SOUTH BEACH DIET COOKBOOK

Most Wanted Recipes With Foolproof Meal Plan for Fast Weight Loss

(Powerful Tips to Lose Weight and Feel Great Forever)

Brandi Bigler

Published by Alex Howard

© Brandi Bigler

All Rights Reserved

South Beach Diet Cookbook: Most Wanted Recipes With Foolproof Meal Plan for Fast Weight Loss (Powerful Tips to Lose Weight and Feel Great Forever)

ISBN 978-1-77485-018-3

All rights reserved. No part of this guide may be reproduced in any form without permission in writing from the publisher except in the case of brief quotations embodied in critical articles or reviews.

Legal & Disclaimer

The information contained in this book is not designed to replace or take the place of any form of medicine or professional medical advice. The information in this book has been provided for educational and entertainment purposes only.

The information contained in this book has been compiled from sources deemed reliable, and it is accurate to the best of the Author's knowledge; however, the Author cannot guarantee its accuracy and validity and cannot be held liable for any errors or omissions. Changes are periodically made to this book. You must consult your doctor or get professional medical advice before using any of the suggested remedies, techniques, or information in this book.

Table of contents

Part 1 1
Introduction 2
What to know about South beach 3
South Beach Diet details 7
What Is the South Beach Diet 8
Purpose 9
How It Works 10
Phase 1: Foods to Include and Foods to Avoid 15
Phases 2 and 3: Foods to Include and Avoid 20
Benefits of the South Beach Diet 23
Downsides of the South Beach Diet 25
Is the South Beach Diet Safe and Sustainable 26
Pros and Cons 27
The South Beach Diet may not be for you 33
HOW DOES THE SOUTH BEACH DIET WORK WITH DIABETES? 34
Why is it popular 34
Risks 35
South beach diet recipe 36
South Beach Diet Meal Plan 36
    Roasted Tomato Breakfast 40

Eggs to go 42

Chile Cheese egg muffins 43

Southern Egg casserole 44

Bacon and Eggs 45

Spinach and cheese bake 46

Ricotta Cream 47

Mango Drink 48

Chocolate Bark 49

Not so mashed potatoes 50

No Pasta Spaghetti 51

Sprout hips 52

Avocado Chicken 53

The best damn salad 54

Cauliflower popcorn 55

Lettuce wraps 56

South Beach Roast 57

Sausage and beans 58

Beef & Beans 59

Greek Vegan 60

Tortilla soup 61

Slow cooker tomato sauce- multipurpose 62

Slow cooked stuffed peppers 63

Taco Soup 64

Dump Cake	65
Conclusion	66
Part 2	69
Hamburger Minestrone Soup	69
Crepes With Ricotta Cocoa Filling	71
Peanut Butter Muffins	73
Muffin	74
Chocolate Meringue Cookies	75
Chocolate Meringue Cookies	76
Lettuce Wrap	77
Cauliflower - Spinach	78
Oven Roasted Vegetables	79
Chicken and Lentil Stew	80
Sausage Veggie Muffins	82
Diet Soup	84
Steak Diane	86
Spaghetti Squash	88
Stuffed Bell Peppers	90
7 - Day - Soup	92
Tiramisu	97
Salmon With Creamy Lemon Sauce Low Carb	99
Sugar Free Peanut Butter Delight	100
Cauliflower Mash With Chives	101

Pepper Crusted Tenderloin of Beef 103

Chicken-Pistachio Salad 105

Thai Shrimp Soup With Lime and Cilantro 107

Mashed Potatoes 109

Cheesy Ham Omelet 110

Pineapple Juice with Rum 111

Pie 112

Haystacks 114

Cola Chicken 115

Cabbage Soup 116

Chocolate Peanut Butter Muffins 117

Chicken Capri 118

Cheerio's Diet Snack 120

Cream of Broccoli Soup 121

Pineapple Muffins 123

Cucumber Water 124

Snickers 125

Coleslaw 127

Chicken Piccata 128

Wasabi-Ginger Glazed Tuna Steaks 130

Tomato Salad 132

Mexican Soup 134

Zucchini Lasagna With Beef and Sausage 136

Blueberry Ginger Mojito Pitchers	139
Wavy Endive, Prosciutto and Mozzarella on Bruschetta	141
Astounding Fried Chicken	143
Smoked Salmon Spread	145
Hawaiian Beef Teriyaki	146
Clam Rocks at the Rib	148
Early lunch Breads	151
Chocolate Chip Walnut Cupcakes	154
Crab and Potato Frittata	156
Long Island Iced Tea	158
Flame broiled Corn on the Cob with BBQ Butter	159
Spaghetti with Summer Squash and Tomatoes	162
Peaches in Sauternes	165
Container Seared Florida Pompano and Spiny Lobster in Squab Consomme, and Poached Foie Gras	166
Chocolate S'mores	171
Meat and Broccoli Salad	173
Swordfish and Spaghetti with Citrus Pesto	175
Brilliant Oven-Roasted Capon	177
Superbly Crunchy Slaw	180
Lemon Shakerato	182
Feline's Broccoli Slaw	182
Container Seared Barramundi with "Caruru"	183

Berries with Spiced Cream 186

Atlantic Beach Pie 187

Flame broiled Mahi-Mahi, Ceviche-Style 189

Part 1

Introduction

The South Beach Diet has been popular for over a decade.

It's a lower-carb diet that has been credited with producing rapid weight loss without hunger, all while promoting heart health.

On the other hand, it's also been criticized for being a restrictive "fad" diet.

This article provides a detailed review of the South Beach Diet, including its benefits, downsides, safety and sustainability.

The South Beach Diet was created in the mid-1990s by Dr. Arthur Agatston, a Florida-based cardiologist. His work in heart disease research led to the development of the Agatston score, which measures the amount of calcium in the coronary arteries.

According to published interviews, Dr. Agatston observed that patients on the Atkins Diet were losing weight and belly fat, while those on low-fat, high-carb diets were struggling to achieve results.

However, he was uncomfortable with the high amount of saturated fat allowed on the Atkins Diet, especially for people with heart disease. In addition, he didn't believe in restricting high-fiber foods with "good carbs," like fruit and whole grains.

Dr. Agatston wanted to create a diet that allowed overweight, diabetic and prediabetic individuals to easily lose weight and reduce their risk of heart disease.

Therefore, he developed the South Beach Diet, which is rich in low-glycemic-index carbs, lean proteins and unsaturated fats.

After losing weight and belly fat when he tried the diet out on himself, he began prescribing it to his patients, who reported similar results.

Dr. Agatston's book The South Beach Diet was published in 2003 and became a bestseller around the world. An updated version called The South Beach Diet Supercharged was published in 2009 and also became a worldwide bestseller.

What to know about South beach

How to Greet Someone

In Miami, you'll probably end up kissing someone you may never see again that's just part of the culture. While most people in the U.S. shake hands upon meeting, kissing someone on the cheeks isn't out-of-bounds. If you're with a host, follow their lead.

Local Tips

• Do get off Miami Beach, and South Beach in particular the city is so much more than Collins Avenue.

• Don't take it personally if someone cuts you off or honks. Miami drivers are aggressive drivers, and you'll have to become one if you want to get around by car (more on that later).

• Do be ready to order food and drinks when your waiter comes by the first time around. Service is notoriously slow in Miami, and will get slower the longer you keep the server waiting.

• Don't step out on a crosswalk or try to cross the street without looking both ways and making sure cars are far away from you. It's not like it is in New York people are slow to stop, and will get dangerously close to hitting you.

• Do learn a few words in Spanish. Miami is unofficially a bilingual city more than 70 percent of its residents are Hispanic and a few phrases are always good to know. Hola, cómo estás? (Hi, how are you?), gracias (thank you), and un cafecito, por favor (a Cuban espresso, please) will help ingratiate you with Spanish-speaking locals.

• Don't expect things to start exactly on time but don't be late, either. That's just rude.

How to Get Around

Miami has the largest street-grid system in the Southeast, and most people get around by car which means traffic is a bit of beast. If you do rent a car, make sure you get a SunPass to pay tolls, and always be prepared to park (Miami and Miami Beach have apps for places you can't pay a meter) and pay dearly: street parking in South Beach will run you, for example. If you think you can let an unpaid meter run, think again: Miami is also notorious for enforcing parking rules, and you will get towed. If you want to skip the rental car and take public transit, be prepared to wait: The Metrobus system is fairly expansive, but because of all that traffic (remember?), the bus is rarely on time. (Get this app to help you see just where it is) . Car2Go and Citi Bike are two sharing services that allow you to register and get around. Trollies are free, and Uber and Lyft are legal. Miami Beach is walkable, as is downtown Miami, but you'll need a car to get between the two.

Beach Etiquette

Though we encourage you to spend some time off the sand, skipping the beach entirely when visiting Miami is like going to Rome and saying, "Nah, forget the Vatican"—you just don't do it. So whether you decide to sunbathe at Bal Harbour Beach or swim on Mid-Beach, follow the same basic rules: Don't plunk down five feet from a neighbor's stretch of sand, even if it is a particularly glorious stretch. Don't shed your suit unless it's actually a "clothing-optional" beach (if you're looking for one, Haulover Beach is one of the best). Don't drink on the beach—it's illegal. Keep the music down, and pick up your trash when you leave. It's worth noting that many hotels like the Faena, The Betsy, and The Setai have their own "private" beaches—really, stretches of sand restricted to hotel guests and their guests. This access isn't free, but it's usually lumped into a mandatory hotel or resort fee that's tacked onto your overnight rate, so you may as well take advantage of it. Private beaches are cleaner and quieter than public ones, and at some, you'll even be able to order food and drinks from the hotel's bar—all without leaving your chair.

What to Wear

Miami's year-round temps tend to stay above 75 degrees, which means you'll rarely need anything warmer than a light jacket. Come evening, ditch the flip-flops and linen dresses: Though things are kept casual on the beach, people here dress up when going out for dinner—think high heels, and white all year round. Many clubs have a dress code, too; you may get stopped at the door if you're in ripped jeans, T-shirts, or tennis shoes (upscale sneakers are fine—just leave the Nikes at home).

South Beach Diet details

The South Beach Diet says that its balance of complex carbs, lean protein and healthy fats makes it a nutrient-dense, fiber-rich diet that you can follow for a lifetime of healthy eating. Food sources of complex carbs, or so-called good carbs, include fruit, vegetables, whole grains, beans and legumes. Simple carbs, or "bad" carbs, include sugar, syrup and baked goods made from refined white flour.

The South Beach Diet also teaches you about the different kinds of dietary fats and encourages you to limit unhealthy fats while eating more foods with healthier monounsaturated fats. The South Beach Diet emphasizes the benefits of fiber and whole grains and encourages you to include fruits and vegetables in your eating plan.

Carbohydrates

The South Beach Diet is lower in carbohydrates than is a typical eating plan, but not as low as a strict low-carb diet. On a typical eating plan, about 45% to 65% of your daily calories come from carbohydrates. Based on a 2,000-calorie-a-day diet, this amounts to about 225 to 325 grams of carbohydrates a day.

In the final maintenance phase of the South Beach Diet, you can get as much as 28% of your daily calories from carbohydrates, or about 140 grams of carbohydrates a day. A strict low-carb diet might restrict your carb intake to as little as 20 to 100 grams a day. The keto version of the South Beach diet limits carbs to 40 grams a day during phase 1, and 50 grams during phase 2.

Exercise

The South Beach Diet has evolved over time and now recommends exercise as an important part of your lifestyle. The South Beach Diet says that regular exercise will boost your metabolism and help prevent weight-loss plateaus

What Is the South Beach Diet

The South Beach Diet was originally a diet plan outlined in a book by Arthur Agatston, MD. The doctor developed the plan in the 1990s to help his patients lose weight. The South Beach Diet: The Delicious, Doctor-Designed, Foolproof Plan for Fast and Healthy Weight Loss flew off shelves in 2003 when it was first published. Dr. Agatston noticed that patients on the Atkins diet were losing weight and abdominal fat. Being a cardiologist, he was concerned by the amount of saturated fat on Atkins, so he developed his own high-protein, low-carb diet that is lower in saturated fat.

Since that time, the book has gone through several variations and changes, but the core of the eating plan has stayed the same. The South Beach Diet is a low-carb, high-protein and low-sugar program.2? The diet is based in part on the glycemic Index, which ranks foods according to glycemic load. As you learn how to do the South Beach Diet, you learn how to choose healthier, lower sugar foods to keep you full and satisfied so you eat less and slim down.

Purpose

The purpose of the South Beach Diet is to change the overall balance of the foods you eat to encourage weight loss and a healthy lifestyle. The South Beach Diet says it's a healthy way of eating whether you want to lose weight or not.

Why you might follow the South Beach Diet

You might choose to follow the South Beach Diet because you:

• Enjoy the types and amounts of food featured in the diet

• Want a diet that restricts certain carbs and fats to help you lose weight

• Want to change your overall eating habits

• Want a diet you can stick with for life

- Like the related South Beach Diet products, such as cookbooks and diet foods

Check with your doctor or dietitian before starting any weight-loss diet, especially if you have any health concerns.

How It Works

This diet focuses on a healthy balance between carbs, protein, and fat. More importantly, you are advised to consume high-quality carbohydrates, lean protein, and healthy fats. Foods with added sugars, like baked goods, sweets, and soft drinks are off limits. So if you are used to filling up on these foods, the diet may be hard to follow. Prepackaged South Beach Diet foods, such as shakes, snack bars and prepared breakfast, lunch, and dinner meals are available for consumers who sign up for the paid program. Many of these foods are similar to foods that you may feel uncomfortable giving up. But you'll eat them in smaller quantities if you buy the South Beach versions and the foods are prepared with fewer calories. The diet has three stages, known as phases, during which the proportion of carbohydrates is gradually increased, while the proportion of fats and protein are simultaneously decreased. The diet is comprised of a list of recommended foods such as lean meats, vegetables, and "good" (mostly monounsaturated) fats. All three phases include specific allowable foods, meal plans, and recipes. Each phase also includes foods to avoid.

The South Beach Diet is now a home-delivery program broken into two phases. There's no counting calories – the bulk of your food shows up at your door. You'll receive three meals a day, plus snacks if you've ordered the "tier 2" program. The diet lasts as long as you want – it depends on your weight-loss goal.

Phase one is the weight-loss phase. You will stay in this phase until you reach your desired weight-loss goal or you want more flexibility in your food choices. In phase one, you will limit daily net carbs to 50 grams. You'll include high-quality protein (such as fish, shellfish, chicken, turkey, lean beef and soy) and nonstarchy vegetables. You may include very small quantities of beans and legumes, and extremely small amounts of high-fiber fruits like berries and high-protein whole grains like quinoa.

You will jumpstart phase one with a "Body Reboot," lasting one week and including three meals and three snacks each day. On most day, you will include South Beach Diet prepared breakfasts, lunches, dinners and two snacks (a bar and a shake.) Twice each week, you will include two DIY meals, which can be cooked at home or eaten out. In addition to South Beach Diet prepared foods, you'll need to purchase some of your own fresh grocery foods to complete the plan. After the Body Reboot week, you will continue on to phase one. Lower-carb alcohol, such as a glass of dry red wine, is OK, but it should be limited to no more than two servings a week.

Phase two, the maintenance phase, is your lifelong healthy way to eat. You'll begin to reintroduce more "good carbs," such as whole grains, low-sugar fruits and starchy vegetables. You'll also begin to increase your daily net carbs with a goal between 75 and 100 grams per day. You'll keep up a high protein intake, representing at least 25% of your daily calories, to maintain muscle mass. Although no food is off-limits, some individuals — such as people who are insulin-resistant or postmenopausal women — may have more success by continuing to limit their carbs. During this phase, you can continue ordering South Beach products a la carte, and you're encouraged to use portion-control containers and the program guide to transition to this stage.

South Beach is launching a keto-friendly diet approach planned for late 2019. The South Beach Keto Diet Friendly plan includes elements of the ketogenic diet — low carbs and high fat — but does not require you to be as strict in limiting your carbohydrate intake, allowing for more variety in the diet. The South Beach Diet Keto Friendly approach does not require you to be or stay in ketosis to see the weight-loss benefits.

South Beach Diet Phase 1 (also called 7-Day Reboot)

For most people, the most difficult part of the program is Phase 1. In some versions of the plan, this phase lasted for two weeks. However, current versions of the use a 7-day "reboot" instead of a two-week phase. This first part of the plan is the most stringent of the three phases. It is when you will limit the most carbs from your daily diet, including fruit, bread, rice, potatoes, pasta, sugar, alcohol, and baked goods. The theory behind this phase is that there is a switch inside us that affects the way our bodies react to the food we eat and makes us gain weight. When the switch is on, we crave foods that actually cause us to store fat. However, by following the specified plan, you can correct the way your body reacts to food. Many South Beach Diet fans swear that their cravings for sweets and other bad carbs virtually disappear during this reboot. For some, the first phase can be extended, but it is not meant to be a permanent way of eating.

Phase 1 lasts 14 days. It's considered the strictest phase because it limits fruit, grains and other higher-carb foods in order to decrease blood sugar and insulin levels, stabilize hunger and reduce cravings. Most people can expect to lose 8–13 pounds (3.5–6 kg) of body weight during this phase. During phase 1, you consume three meals per day composed of lean protein, non-starchy vegetables and small amounts of healthy fat and legumes. In addition, you consume two mandatory snacks per day, preferably a combination of lean protein and vegetables.

South Beach Diet Phase 2

During this phase, you can start adding in more foods, such as additional sources of carbohydrates, like beans and legumes. During Phase 2, the calorie range and the macronutrient breakdown are almost the same as in Phase 1 but the number of calories allowed from saturated fats decreases to less than 10 percent of total calories. The exercise recommendation is to engage in at least 30 minutes of physical activity each day. Beginning in Phase 2 you can engage in more intense physical activity, if desired.

This phase begins on day 15 and should be maintained for as many weeks as necessary to achieve your goal weight. You can expect to lose 1–2 pounds (0.5–1 kg) per week during this phase, on average. During phase 2, all foods from phase 1 are allowed, plus limited portions of fruit and "good carbs," such as whole grains and certain types of alcohol.

South Beach Diet Phase 3

Phase 3 is the final and least restrictive part of The South Beach Diet.2? Dr. Agatston says as long as you continue to follow some basic guidelines, the diet becomes your way of life and you'll continue to maintain your weight.

Once you achieve your target weight, you advance to phase three. In this stage, although the phase-2 guidelines should be the basis for your lifestyle, occasional treats are allowed and no foods are truly off limits. However, if you overindulge and start putting on weight, Dr. Agatston recommends returning to phase 1 for one to two weeks before returning to phase three. In The South Beach Diet Supercharged, Dr. Agatston also recommends regular exercise and provides a three-phase fitness program to accompany the diet phases.

Phase 1: Foods to Include and Foods to Avoid

Foods to Include

Please note that the guidelines for all phases are from the book, The South Beach Diet Supercharged. The guidelines on the South Beach Diet website may be different.

Lean Protein

Although portions aren't limited, the diet recommends slowly consuming a small portion and returning for seconds if you are still hungry.

- Lean beef, pork, lamb, veal and game
- Skinless chicken and turkey breast
- Fish and shellfish
- Turkey bacon and pepperoni
- Eggs and egg whites
- Soy-based meat substitutes
- Low-fat hard cheese, ricotta cheese and cottage cheese
- Buttermilk, low-fat milk, plain or Greek yogurt, kefir and soy milk, limited to 2 cups (473 ml) daily

Non-Starchy Vegetables

Consume a minimum of 4 1/2 cups daily. All vegetables are allowed except beets, carrots, corn, turnips, yams, peas, white potatoes and most types of winter squash.

Legumes

Limit these to 1/3–1/2 cup per day, cooked, unless otherwise noted.

- Black beans, kidney beans, pinto beans, navy beans, garbanzo beans and other bean varieties

- Split peas and black-eyed peas

- Lentils

- Edamame and soybeans

- Hummus, limited to 1/4 cup

- Nuts and Seeds

- Limit these to 1 oz (28 grams) per day.

- Almonds, cashews, macadamias, pecans, pistachios, walnuts and other nuts

- Nut butters, limited to 2 tbsp

- Flaxseeds, chia seeds, sesame seeds, pumpkin seeds and other seeds

Oils and Fats

Limited to 2 tbsp of oil per day. Monounsaturated oils are encouraged.

- Monounsaturated oils, such as olive, canola, macadamia and avocado oils

- Vegetable and seed oils, such as corn, flaxseed, grapeseed, peanut, safflower, sesame and soybean oil

- Alternative Fat Choices

- Each serving is equivalent to 2 tbsp of healthy oils.

- Avocado, limited to 2/3 of one fruit
- Trans-fat-free margarine, limited to 2 tbsp
- Low-fat mayonnaise, limited to 2 tbsp
- Regular mayonnaise, limited to 1 tbsp
- Salad dressing with less than 3 grams sugar, limited to 2 tbsp
- Olives, limited to 20–30, depending on size

Sweet Treats

Limit consumption to 100 calories or fewer per day.

- Sugar-free or unsweetened cocoa or chocolate syrup
- Sugar-free gelatin, jams and jellies
- Sugar-free candies, popsicles or gum
- Sugar substitutes, including Stevia, artificial sweeteners and sugar alcohols like xylitol and erythritol

Broth

- Herbs, spices, horseradish, mustard, lemon juice or salsa
- All vinegars, with balsamic limited to 1 tbsp
- Light coconut milk, limited 1/4 cup (59 ml)

- Soy sauce, steak sauce or miso, limited to 1 1/2 tsp (7 ml)
- Cream, whole milk or half and half, limited to 1 tbsp
- Light sour cream or cream cheese, limited to 2 tbsp
- Light whipped topping, limited to 2 tbsp

Beverages

You may drink unlimited quantities of these beverages, although drinking your caffeine in moderation is advised.

- Coffee, regular or decaffeinated
- Tea, regular, decaffeinated or herbal
- Sugar-free sodas
- Sugar-free drink mixes
- Tomato juice or vegetable juice

Foods to Avoid

Certain fatty foods and those high in carbs, including fruits and grains, are not allowed in phase 1. These include:

- Fatty meat and poultry

- Butter and coconut oil
- Whole milk
- Foods made with refined sugar
- Honey, maple syrup and agave nectar
- Grains
- All fruits and fruit juice
- Beets, carrots, corn, turnips, yams, peas, white potatoes and winter squash
- Alcohol

Phases 2 and 3: Foods to Include and Avoid

Foods to Include

Phase 2 includes all phase 1 foods and gradually adds in higher-carb foods, beginning with one daily serving of fruit and whole grains or starchy vegetables for the first week. On the 14th day of phase 2 and thereafter, you may consume up to three servings of fruit and four servings of whole grains and starchy vegetables per day. An occasional alcoholic drink is also allowed, although choices are limited to light beer and dry wine. Once you've achieved your goal weight, you move to phase three for maintenance. During this phase, you should generally follow the guidelines from phase 2.

However, you can include "treat" foods occasionally, since no foods are completely off limits.

Fruits

Consume 1–3 servings per day. All fresh and frozen fruits are allowed except dates, figs, pineapple, raisins and watermelon. A serving size is one small piece of fruit, half a grapefruit or 3/4 cup (about 115 grams) berries, cherries or grapes.

Whole Grains and Starchy Vegetables

Consume 1–4 servings per day.

Except where noted, one serving size is 1/2 cup cooked starchy vegetables, 1 slice bread or 1/2 cup cooked grains.

- Peas
- Rutabaga
- Sweet potatoes and yams
- Turnips
- Winter squash, limited to 3/4 cup
- Whole-grain hot cereal

- Whole-grain cold cereal, limited to 1 cup
- Whole-grain bread
- Brown or wild rice
- Whole-grain pasta, quinoa, couscous or farro
- Taro, limited to 1/3 cup
- Popcorn, limited to 3 cups
- Whole-grain bagel, limited to 1/2 small
- Pita bread, limited to 1/2 pita
- Corn or whole-grain tortilla, limited to 1 small

Alcohol

- One daily serving of dry wine or an occasional light beer is allowed.
- Light beer, limited to 12 oz (355 ml)
- Wine, dry red or white, limited to 4 oz (118 ml)

Phases 2 and 3: Foods to Avoid

Phase 2 of the South Beach Diet discourages intake of fatty meats, saturated fat and foods high in refined or natural sugar. Try to avoid:

- Fatty meat and poultry

- Butter and coconut oil
- Whole milk
- Foods made with refined flour or sugar
- Honey, maple syrup, agave nectar
- Fruit juice
- Beets, corn and white potatoes
- Dates, figs, pineapple, raisins and watermelon
- Alcohol other than light beer and dry wine

Benefits of the South Beach Diet

There are several benefits of the South Beach diet, including its ability to produce weight loss without hunger.Research, including an analysis of 24 studies, has consistently shown that high-protein, low-carb diets are effective for weight loss. Part of this is due to protein's ability to increase your metabolic rate. In addition, protein helps modify hormone levels that reduce hunger and promote fullness, so you end up naturally eating less

What's more, gradually adding small amounts of healthy carbs back into your diet may promote continued weight loss in some people and make it easier for them to stick to the diet long-term. In one study, overweight and obese people with metabolic syndrome followed the South Beach Diet for 12 weeks. By the end of the study, they had lost 11 pounds (5.2 kg) and 2 inches (5.1 cm) from around their waists, on average. They also experienced significant decreases in fasting insulin and an increase in the fullness hormone CCK. The South Beach Diet encourages a high intake of fatty fish like salmon and other foods that fight inflammation, such as leafy greens and cruciferous veggies. In addition, it recommends dieters regularly consume eggs, nuts, seeds, extra virgin olive oil and other foods that have been shown to protect heart health.

Research published in 2019 suggests that a low-carb diet may help people who:

• wish to lose weight quickly in the early stages

• have type 2 diabetes and need to control their blood sugar levels

However, it remains unclear whether it will help to manage cardiovascular risk. Some studies have found that low-density lipoprotein (LDL) cholesterol rose when a person followed a low-carb diet, but others have found only small changes. The creators of the diet list several advantages of their approach.

They say that people who follow the diet are better able to:

• maintain an ideal body weight for the long term

- avoid diabetes

- achieve normal cholesterol and blood fat levels

- prevent hypertension

The South Beach Diet, they say, means that people enjoy better health and feel satisfied with the food they eat. The approach offers a lifestyle, rather than a diet.

Downsides of the South Beach Diet

Unfortunately, the South Beach Diet also has a couple of drawbacks. The main issue is that it may be overly restrictive with respect to the amounts and types of fats allowed. In addition, it allows potentially harmful types of fat, such as soybean oil and safflower oil, which are extremely high in omega-6 fatty acids. Although it's important to get some omega-6 fats in your diet, if you're like most people, you probably already get far more than you need. In contrast, if you eat a Western Diet, it's likely you get too little of the anti-inflammatory omega-3 fats found in fatty fish like salmon, sardines and mackerel. Consuming a high ratio of omega-6 to omega-3 fats has been linked to inflammation, heart disease and other health problems.

In contrast, butter and coconut oil aren't included on the South Beach Diet because they are high in saturated fat. However, coconut oil has been credited with several health benefits, including weight loss, a reduction in belly fat and better heart health markers in overweight and obese adults. In addition, most comprehensive reviews of studies have found no association between saturated fat intake and an increased risk of heart disease. On the other hand, other large reviews have found that replacing a portion of saturated fat with unsaturated fat could potentially reduce the risk of heart disease. Overall, choosing less processed fat and eating plenty of fish high in omega-3 fats may be more important for heart health than restricting saturated fat.

Is the South Beach Diet Safe and Sustainable

The South Beach Diet is a healthy way of eating that is far lower in carbs than conventional low-fat diets. It also encourages dieters to eat mainly unprocessed foods, liberal amounts of vegetables and healthy, high-fiber carb sources. However, the diet allows processed vegetable oils, which could pose health risks. Nevertheless, you can avoid this drawback by choosing unprocessed monounsaturated fats like extra virgin olive oil, avocado oil or macadamia oil instead. All this being said, the South Beach Diet is likely a sustainable way of eating. Many people have reported losing weight and keeping it off by following the diet. Yet in the end, the most effective diet for weight loss is whichever one you can easily stick with long-term.

Pros and Cons

Like any diet, the South Beach Diet has its own set of positives and negatives. On the upside, the South Beach Diet is super simple and it encourages individual experimentation. When you sign up for the paid version of the program, you won't have to do any guesswork about portion sizes, and whether or not you pay for the program, the allowed and not allowed foods are clearly outlined. On the other hand, the first portion of the South Beach Diet can seem extremely restrictive and potentially lead to disordered eating or yo-yo dieting down the road. Additionally, this diet promotes consumption of processed, packaged foods (the bars and shakes that come with the plan). The South Beach Diet may also not be structured enough in the later phases, which could result in weight regain for people who aren't sure how to control portion sizes after phases 1 and 2. The South Beach Diet has been popular for over a decade. It's a lower-carb diet that has been credited with producing rapid weight loss without hunger, all while promoting heart health. On the other hand, it's also been criticized for being a restrictive "fad" diet. This article provides a detailed review of the South Beach Diet, including its benefits, downsides, safety and sustainability.

The South Beach Diet was created in the mid-1990s by Dr. Arthur Agatston, a Florida-based cardiologist. His work in heart disease research led to the development of the Agatston score, which measures the amount of calcium in the coronary arteries. According to published interviews, Dr. Agatston observed that patients on the Atkins Diet were losing weight and belly fat, while those on low-fat, high-carb diets were struggling to achieve results. However, he was uncomfortable with the high amount of saturated fat allowed on the Atkins Diet, especially for people with heart disease. In addition, he didn't believe in restricting high-fiber foods with "good carbs," like fruit and whole grains. Dr. Agatston wanted to create a diet that allowed overweight, diabetic and prediabetic individuals to easily lose weight and reduce their risk of heart disease. Therefore, he developed the South Beach Diet, which is rich in low-glycemic-index carbs, lean proteins and unsaturated fats. After losing weight and belly fat when he tried the diet out on himself, he began prescribing it to his patients, who reported similar results.

Dr. Agatston's book The South Beach Diet was published in 2003 and became a bestseller around the world. An updated version called The South Beach Diet Supercharged was published in 2009 and also became a worldwide bestseller. The South Beach Diet has three different phases: two for weight loss and a third for weight maintenance.

The South Beach Diet is a popular diet that takes you through phases. During Phase 1, you'll cut out virtually all carbohydrates to get rid of bloat and "reboot" your body; during Phase 2, you'll slowly start adding carbohydrates back into your body; and by Phase 3, you're expected to have met your goal weight and learned new healthy eating habits. The South Beach Diet claims to make you feel less hungry and contribute to a number of good health outcomes, including lower triglycerides and blood glucose; lower blood pressure, higher HDL, among others. But like all diets, not everyone takes well to the South Beach Diet. Here we explain the positives and negatives of the diet and what sets it apart from other low-carb diets.

Pros of the South Beach Diet

Overall, the South Beach Diet can be healthy and well-rounded, with the exception of the first phase, which restricts carbohydrate intake.

Simplicity

There's no counting and not much measuring on the South Beach Diet. For the most part, you just choose foods from certain lists and eat within that, so you won't have to deal with any guesswork or counting calories of each food.

Low in Saturated Fats

Low-carb diet authors have different opinions on whether it's important to limit saturated fats on reduced carb diets; however, no author recommends relying on them.

Encourages Individual Experimentation

One of the strongest aspects of the diet is the focus on each person being aware of the effects of foods on their bodies, particularly as they add carbohydrates. Using the marker of carb cravings can be a useful one, as it's vital for people who are sensitive to carbohydrates to be aware of what foods and what quantities trigger these cravings.

Gives Your Body a Chance to Reset

While we don't think fasting or restricting food groups is the best way to start any healthy eating program, a one-week reset does work well for many people. For example, you may have some food sensitivities you didn't know about, and Phase 1 of the South Beach Diet could help you uncover those.

Emphasizes Healthy Eating Patterns

After Phase 1 ends, the South Beach Diet is really all about creating sustainable and well-rounded eating patterns. The end goal does involve weight loss for most people, but South Beach emphasizes long-term healthy habits, and that's a goal we can get behind. A successful version of the South Beach Diet involves powering through the first phase and then slowly discovering how many carbohydrates (and what kinds) your body can handle. The South Beach Diet offers some positives that make it a great diet for some (e.g., those who value simplicity) but may not be the best choice for everyone.

Cons of the South Beach Diet

Like most diets, the South Beach Diet presents some drawbacks, most of which revolve around its restrictive and difficult Phase 1.

Very Restrictive First Phase

The limitations of the first phase may be a real turn off for some people. On the other hand, it's short-term, and the author doesn't recommend anyone staying with it longer than 3 or 4 weeks at most (for people who have quite a bit of weight to lose). Since there are no guidelines as to how much carbohydrate to eat, "carb crash" could also occur, depending upon the individual dieter's food selections.

Some Inconsistencies

Quite a few aspects of the diet don't really fit together well. For example, more saturated fat is allowed in Phase 3, when a primary aspect in Phases 1 and 2 was to limit saturated fat. Additionally, the creator, Dr. Aruthur Agatston recommends some highly processed carbs, such as couscous, and has many recipes which include it. Other high-glycemic foods are in his menus and recipes, which may send, at the least, a mixed message.

No Evidence for Weight Loss

The South Beach Diet markets itself as a weight-loss solution, but there's no solid evidence to uphold that claim. According to a study published in 2016, there is evidence that low-carb diets support weight loss, but South Beach doesn't stay low-carb for long, so that relationship doesn't pan out, either. There is little research on the South Beach diet, however a study published in 2014 suggested that it isn't any more effective than other commercial diets, and is especially ineffective at promoting long-term weight loss.

Possibly Not Enough Structure

For some people, there may not be enough structure when it comes to adding carbs back in. This diet leaves a lot up to the individual, which is good in the long run but is probably harder in the short run. Also, some people just aren't all that tuned into their bodies' signals and might not be motivated to become so.

Can Be Expensive

You can follow the South Beach principles on your own, but if you opt to participate in the paid program and get meals delivered to your door, expect to pay a few hundred dollars per month for the convenience.

May Contribute to Disordered Eating

Any diet that labels foods as "good" and "bad" hold the potential to result in disordered eating and an unhealthy relationship with food. Because the South Beach Diet places such an emphasis on "good" and "bad" carbohydrate sources and fats, it may lead to food fear. In the end, whether or not you should try the South Beach Diet comes down to personal preference and your goals. You should start a diet for the right reasons, and South Beach might be right for you if:

• You want to uncover food sensitivities to carbohydrate sources

• You want a one-week "reboot" that may help you feel better without too severely restricting calorie intake

• You want to learn more about your body and what a healthy eating pattern looks like for you

The South Beach Diet may not be for you

If:

- You're solely in it for weight loss (there's no solid evidence to support this)

- You have a history of disordered eating or an unhealthy relationship with food or your body

- You're very active: lack of carbohydrates may affect your athletic performance or lead to hypoglycemia

HOW DOES THE SOUTH BEACH DIET WORK WITH DIABETES?

Like the Atkins Diet, the South Beach diet takes place in phases. As well as carbohydrates, the South Beach diet also restricts saturated fats.

The carbohydrate limitations of the South Beach Diet also allow more carbohydrates than an Atkins diet The South Beach diet makes a distinction between good and bad carbohydrates, and excludes the latter.

Why is it popular

The creators of the diet say that people choose it because it is an effective and flexible way of losing weight, without having to count calories. Part of its popularity might be that it helps people to change overall eating habits, and because there are cook books and diet food products that accompany it.

Risks

The South Beach Diet is popular, but people should approach all lifestyle changes with caution.

Low carbohydrates

Restricting carbohydrates too much can lead to ketosis. This is a potentially serious health problem in which substances known as ketones build up in the body as the body burns fat for energy.

Lack of supporting evidence

In 2006, three years after the South Beach Diet book appeared, research published in the Journal of General Internal Medicine suggested that up to 67 percent of the "facts" stated in it may not have scientific evidence to support them. Some of the health claims and "facts" that were disproven or not supported by an exhaustive medical review of evidence include:

- "People lose 8 to 13 pounds in the first 2 weeks."

- "Carrots, beets, and watermelon promote weight gain because of a high GI (glycemic index)."

- "Fats and protein cause satiety more efficiently than carbohydrates."

- "This diet (South Beach) has been scientifically studied and proven effective."

Experts recommend being skeptical of popular diets' health guarantees.

South beach diet recipe
What types of meals should you eat on South Beach Diet

South Beach moves through three phases. Phase one lasts two weeks: lots of lean protein, vegetables, salads, beans, eggs, low-fat dairy and a bit of healthy fats, such as nuts and olive oil. No fruit, starches (pasta, rice or bread), whole grains, sugary foods or alcohol. Phase two brings back "good" carbs like whole-grain bread, brown rice, whole-wheat pasta and fruit (and a glass of wine with dinner). When you hit your weight goal and enter phase three, no food is off-limits. There are still rules, however, among them no more than 2 tablespoons of fat, such as mayonnaise or margarine, a day.

South Beach Diet Meal Plan

Here's a day of typical meals in phases one and two. During phase one, you eat five times per day three meals and two snacks. All meals and snacks (including shakes and a dark chocolate nut bar) are provided, but you'll need to add in at five servings of fresh non-starchy vegetables and 64 ounces of water each day. During phase two, you'll eat more often and include more starchy vegetables, "good" carbohydrates and DIY meals.

Phase One: One-Week Body Reboot

Breakfast

South Beach Diet tropical coconut almond bar

Morning snack

South Beach complete shake

- 1 serving of non-starchy vegetables

Lunch

South Beach Diet chicken roma

- 2 servings of non-starchy vegetables

Afternoon snack

South Beach Diet dark chocolate nut bar

Dinner

South Beach Diet taqueria-style beef and cheese skillet

- 2 servings of non-starchy vegetables

Phase: Week 2 and Beyond (Women)

Breakfast

- 1 large egg
- 1/2 avocado

Morning snack

- Greek yogurt, full-fat, 5.3 ounces

Lunch

- 2 ounces deli turkey
- 1 tbsp olive-oil based mayo
- 1 slice whole-grain bread

Afternoon snack

- 1 medium orange

Dinner

- 3 ounces pork tenderloin

- 1/2 cup olives
- 1/2 cup cooked whole-wheat pasta

Evening Snack

- 1 ounce cheddar cheese

Phase: Week 2 and Beyond (Men)

Breakfast

- 2 large eggs
- 1/2 avocado

Morning snack

- Greek yogurt, full-fat, 5.3 ounces
- 1/4 cup almonds

Lunch

- 2 ounces deli turkey
- 1 tbsp olive-oil based mayo
- 1 slice whole-grain bread

Afternoon snack

- 1 medium orange

Dinner

- 3 ounces pork tenderloin
- 1/2 cup olives
- 1/2 cup cooked whole-wheat pasta

Evening Snack

- 1 ounce cheddar cheese

Roasted Tomato Breakfast

Ingredients:

- 1 Green pepper, sliced
- Nonstick spray
- ½ tsp dried oregano
- 1 C cherry tomatoes, sliced
- ¾ C feta cheese
- 1 dozen eggs
- Salt and pepper to taste

Directions: Set your oven to 350 degrees, grease 9x9 baking dish. Add peppers and spices to dish and bake for about 20 minutes. While that is baking you can start cutting your tomato and beat the eggs in a bowl and spice. After 10 minutes you can add the tomatoes to the peppers. Set the dish back in the oven for about 15 more minutes. Sprinkle Feta cheese over peppers and tomatoes and add eggs over the top of Feta. Now you can add this back to the oven for another 30 minutes or so.

Eggs to go

Ingredients:

- 1 dozen eggs
- 2 tsp all season
- 1 C low fat cheese
- 1-2 diced onions

Directions: Start with preheating your oven to 375 degrees, you want to grease down a muffin tin, you are going to layer everything, ending with the cheese in the middle and on top. Leave enough room at the top for the muffins to rise. You will pour the egg mix around the rest of the ingredients in the muffin tin. So the egg will be the shell for your breakfast muffin. Bake 25 minutes or so, and remove and let cool. You can freeze this, and simply heat for 1-2 minutes in the morning, and you're good to go.

Chile Cheese egg muffins

Ingredients:

- One dozen eggs
- 4 oz. diced chills
- 1 ½ C grated low fat cheese
- 2 T half and half
- Salt and Pepper to taste

Directions: Set oven to 350 degrees, Spray muffin tins, Break eggs in bowl, add half and half, add everything else, and pour mixture into muffin tins and bale for 35 minutes or so at 375 degrees.

Southern Egg casserole

Ingredients:

- 1 ½ dozen eggs
- 1 can chilies
- 14 oz. diced tomatoes
- 1 C shredded cheese
- 3 T diced onions
- Salsa, as garnish

Directions: Preheat oven to 350 degrees, while that is preheating open cans and drain excess liquids. Add cheese to bottom of baking dish add green onions, then eggs. Bake uncovered for about 45 minutes, then remove dish and sprinkle cheese over top, and set back in oven for about 15 minutes. This can be frozen, and recooked later, or you can eat right away.

Bacon and Eggs

Ingredients:

- 1 lbs. chopped, frozen spinach
- 6 slices bread, no crust
- 4 eggs
- 1 ½ C skim milk
- ½ C ketchup
- ½ tsp mace
- ½ C shredded cheese
- ¼ C bacon bits

Directions: You can cook the frozen spinach according to the box/bag. Set this aside you will need it later. Spray down your baking dish and break the bread apart throughout the bottom of the dish. You want one single layer. Whisk your eggs together, adding milk, ketchup, and seasonings. Make sure this is well mixed, and whisked. Add the spinach over the bread, than add the egg mixture over the spinach. Add cheese, by sprinkling over the eggs. Cover and refrigerate until morning. Bake at 350 for 35 minutes in the morning.

Spinach and cheese bake

Ingredients:

- 4 C spinach
- 1-2 tsp olive oil
- 1 ½ C low fat mozzarella
- 1/3 C sliced green onions
- 8 eggs, beaten
- 1 tsp. seasoning
- Salt and pepper to taste

Directions: Preheat your oven to 375 degrees. Spray your baking dish. Add spinach and oil to frying pan until the greens are wilted. Move the spinach to the baking dish and add the eggs, seasoning (need to beaten in a bowl first) to the spinach baking dish. Add cheese over top and bake covered for 35 minutes. This can be frozen and reheated later, or you can serve hot.

Ricotta Cream

Ingredients:

- ½ C skim ricotta
- ½ tsp unsweetened cocoa powder
- ¼ tsp vanilla extract
- 1 package Truvia
- 1 tsp espresso powder
- 5 chocolate chips

Directions: Mix everything together, other than the 5 chocolate chips, that's for the top. Makes a great diet dessert.

Mango Drink

Ingredients:

- Mango
- 1 ½ C yogurt
- 1 T sugar

Directions: You will add everything in a blender, and few ice chips or cold water. You want to puree this in your blender. Serve over ice.

Chocolate Bark

Ingredients:

- 12 oz. chocolate chips
- C pistachio nuts

Directions: Melt the chocolate chips in the microwave generally for about 2 minutes. Add the nuts in, then lay parchment paper over baking sheet, and spoon the chocolate into parchment paper, onto a flat "sheet" like, then add to the fridge for little over an hour. You want this to look like wax chocolate bark. Break this a part and enjoy. Needs to stay refrigerated.

Not so mashed potatoes

Ingredients:

- Cauliflower cut into florets
- 2 T extra virgin olive oil
- 1 T minced garlic
- ¼ C grated parmesan
- 1 T cream cheese (Fat free of course)
- ½ tsp salt to taste
- 1/8 tsp pepper to taste

Directions: Steam cauliflower over saucepan with water. Cover and steam, roughly about 10 minutes. Heat oil in a small skillet and cook garlic until its smooth and you can transfer cauliflower (half of it) to a food processor and blend. Add one more each time until it's all creamy. Blend everything until its smooth.

No Pasta Spaghetti

Ingredients:

- 1 lbs. squash spaghetti
- 1 T extra virgin olive oil
- ½ onion sliced
- ½ zucchini sliced
- 1/8 tsp pepper
- ¼ parmesan

Directions: Slice squash in half face side down and add to baking dish, with 1/8 C water. Set in microwave for 10minutes. In a large skillet add 1 T oil, and sauté onions, add the zucchini and let them brown. Slowly add the remaining ingredients and let it all simmer. Slowly add the strands to a bowl, when done drizzle with oil and parmesan if you wish.

Sprout hips

Ingredients:

- 10-12 Brussels sprouts
- 1 T olive oil
- ¼ tsp salt

Directions: Preheat your oven to 350 degrees, and cut the top off of each of your sprouts, Keep doing this until all the leaves have fallen off. Toss with oil, and lay over baking sheet. Season with salt and roast for roughly 7-10 minutes or until they are crispy, like chips

Avocado Chicken

Ingredients:

- 1 large avocado, chopped
- 1 jalapeno, chopped
- ½ tsp cilantro
- 1 ½ lbs. sliced chicken breast
- 1 tsp. coconut oil

Directions: If everything isn't already chopped, you want to chop the vegetables, and set in a bowl, you can squeeze fresh lemon juice on them if you want, for added flavor. Heat the oil and chicken in a skillet on low, you can season both sides of chicken while cooking, this will generally take about 4-5 minutes on both sides. You can serve the chicken with the avocado.

The best damn salad

Ingredients:

- 2 C cooked chicken
- 1 C diced celery
- 1 C green onlives1
- ½ C sliced green onions
- 1/3 C mayo
- 1/3 C L Miracle whip
- 1 tsp. Dijon
- 1 tsp. celery seed

Directions: If your chicken is already cooked and cooked or shredded, go ahead and add everything together, stir in mayo and miracle whip, and whisk everything else together. Serve cool or warm. Great either way.

Cauliflower popcorn

Ingredients:

- Cauliflower head
- 1 T extra virgin olive oil
- 1 T yeast powder
- ½ tsp salt
- ¼ tsp paprika
- ¼ tsp mustard powder
- ¼ tsp pepper

Directions: Start with preheating oven to 425 degrees and line baking sheet with parchment paper. In bowl you want to toss the florets with other ingredients, Roast for 25 minutes or so. You want to serve this warm.

Lettuce wraps

Ingredients:

- 1 lbs. skinless chicken breasts
- 1 C salsa
- 2 tsp. onion powder
- 1can green chilies
- 1 T hot sauce
- 1 T fresh lime juice
- 2 avocados diced
- 2/4 C chopped cilantro
- 1/4 C onion, diced onion
- ¼ C lime juice
- 2 Large heads of lettuce

Directions: there are ingredients here for the chicken, to be slow cooked, and the salsa that will be served with the wrap add first 6 ingredients together and add to slow cooker for about 2-4 hours on low. The lettuce will serve as your warp bowl. Remove the first 2-3 layers of the lettuce leaving t in the bowl shape. Make salsa while chicken is cooking. This is a great make ahead of time take to work lunch.

South Beach Roast

Ingredients:

- 4-5 lbs. roast
- 1 T steak rub
- 1 T olive oil
- ¼ C water
- 2 onions, sliced
- 1 C beef stock
- ½ C balsamic vinegar
- ½ C tomato sauce

Directions: You want to start taking the fat off, you can trim that off easily if it is thawed. This is your traditional roast, with added flavor and less calories. Add everything together, and cook on low for 6-8 hours or for 4-6 hours on high.

Sausage and beans

Ingredients:

- 1 C dried beans (Canned beans is fine)
- ½ tsp garlic powder
- ½ tsp onion powder
- 5 links Italians sausage
- 1 tsp oil
- 1 bunch greens
- ½ C liquid from canned beans
- 1 tsp. minced garlic

Directions: You want to start with the beans, water and the seasoning. Let this cook for about30 minutes. You just want the beans to be cooked properly. Once cooked drain and save part of the water. Cook the sausage and cut into bite size pieces. Add everything in the slow cooker, and cook on low for 4-6 hours. You can garnish with parmesan cheese if you would like.

Beef & Beans

Ingredients:

- 1 lbs. ground beef
- 1 C chopped onion
- 3 tsp olive oil, separated
- 2 T minced garlic
- 2 tsp. Chile powder
- 2 T ground pepper
- 1 tsp Mexican oregano
- 1 ¼ C salsa
- 1 can pinto beans
- 1 can kidney beans
- 1 can refried beans
- 1 C beef broth
- 2 T lime juice

Directions: Start with 2 tsp of the oil and start your frying pan, add the beef and onions, you want to cook this until it's done. Once this is done, add to slow cooker, add spices to slow cooker along with remaining ingredients, except for refried beans and salsa. Let cook on low for 6-8 hours. Add salsa and refried beans when serving.

Greek Vegan

Ingredients:

- 2 C lentils
- 8 C chicken broth
- 1 onion diced
- 1 C shopped celery
- 1 T seasoning
- 1 tsp thyme
- 1 T minced garlic
- 1 can petite tomatoes and juice
- 1 bunch spinach
- 2 T lemon juice

Directions: Once everything is cleaned or chopped add to slow cooker and set for 4-6 hours on high or 6-8 hours on low.

Tortilla soup

Ingredients:

- 2 cans diced tomatoes
- 2 can green chilies
- 1 onion diced
- 1 bell pepper diced
- 1 box chicken broth
- Garnishes

    Directions" Combine everything in slow cooker other than your garnishes, cook for 4-6 hours on high or longer on low. Serve in bowl, topped with your favorite fat free garnishes, cheese, sour cream etc.

Slow cooker tomato sauce- multipurpose

Ingredients:

- 2 cans diced tomatoes
- 1 onion chopped
- 1 carrot sliced
- 2 celery stalks, chopped

Directions: Combine everything and cook overnight on low. Add pepper flakes as needed or so desire.

Slow cooked stuffed peppers

Ingredients:

- 4 peppers, removed tops and seeded
- 1 lbs. cooked ground sausage
- 2 eggs, beaten
- 1 T minced garlic
- 1/3 C parsley, chopped
- ½ tsp salt
- ½ tsp pepper to taste
- 1 C no sugar pasta sauce

Direction: Make sure peppers are gutted, set slow cooker to low, mix everything else in separate bowl and spoon into each pepper, and add a little water to the bottom of slow cooker, to keep from burning bottoms of peppers. Set on low for 4-5 hours.

Taco Soup

Ingredients:

- 2 lbs. ground beef cooked and set aside
- 1 can diced tomatoes and chilies
- 1 can beef broth
- Shredded cheese
- 1 package taco seasoning

Directions: add 1 T and taco seasoning to cooked ground beef, and add to slow cooker, add remaining ingredients, other than garnishes, set on low for 4-6 hours. Garnish with toppings including cheese as you serve.

Dump Cake

Ingredients:

- Fat free chocolate cake mix
- Low fat instant pudding
- Semi-sweet chocolate chips

Directions: Set slow cooker on low, follow cake mix on box and dump into slow cooker. Add prepared instant pudding in middle of cake mix and set on low for 2-4 hours.

Conclusion

The South Beach Diet is a good weight loss option for those who value convenience and weight loss results above menu freedom. In fact, a lot of women and men who join have already tried the DIY diets and weight loss apps without success. However, no single diet will work for everyone. That's why it's important to do your homework and decide whether the program is a good fit for your lifestyle, personality, and weight loss goals. South Beach claims Phase 1 usually results in weight loss of around eight to thirteen pounds, and Phase 2 results in one to two pounds lost a week. These both make sense, intuitively. Periods of severe carbohydrate restriction are generally accompanied by dramatic short-term weight loss (mainly from water, but some short-term fat loss is definitely accelerated with such a great degree of restriction). Likewise, the cutting out of sugary junk foods, liquid calories, and unhealthy snacking habits and substitution with high-fiber, high-protein options that increase satiety and enhance weight loss efforts seen in Phase 2 will absolutely have a dramatic impact on caloric intake, even in the absence of conscientious counting. This diet is advertised like typical commercial diets, and I do not exactly approve of this, but when you are operating in a market where your customers want to hear anything but the hard truth about losing weight (that it requires eating less and exercising more), you have to do what you have to do.

Phase 1 does put me on high alert. I fail to see how cutting out all alcohol and carbs, even for just two weeks, is going to eliminate cravings. If anything, I would think cravings would increase, to the point that you risk having people go into Phase 2 dying to stuff an entire large pizza down their gullet. I understand a change of pace is desperately needed in individuals used to such unhealthy eating habits, but there are better ways around this (like slowly transitioning into something like Phase 2. That aside, I do want to praise the fact that they emphasize everything in moderation and transitioning into a healthy long-term diet. Weight regain is a humongous issue with commercial diets, so the fact that they not only account for this but actively base their recommendations on what is sustainable in the long run is huge, to me at least. My final words on the matter would be that I can see this being a great option in non-diabetic, overweight individuals looking to drop fat and reduce risk markers associated with excessive weight. I do not at all think counting calories is too much to ask of people, but this definitely appears to be the next best thing.

The South Beach Diet is generally safe if you follow it as outlined in official South Beach Diet books and websites. However, if you severely restrict your carbohydrates, you may experience problems from ketosis. Ketosis occurs when you don't have enough sugar (glucose) for energy, so your body breaks down stored fat, causing ketones to build up in your body. Side effects from ketosis can include nausea, headache, mental fatigue and bad breath, and sometimes dehydration and dizziness

Part 2

Hamburger Minestrone Soup

INGREDIENTS

1 lb extra lean ground beef (less than 10% fat)
1 medium onion, chopped
1 quart reduced-sodium fat-free beef broth
6 cups water
1 (14 1/2 ounce) can diced tomatoes with juice, undrained (no sugar added)
2 cups finely shredded cabbage (I use bagged coleslaw salad mix to save time)
2 stalks celery, diced
1 (15 ounce) can kidney beans, rinsed and drained (or canneloni or great northern beans, no sugar added)
2 tablespoons italian seasoning
1 -2 garlic clove, minced
salt & pepper
parmesan cheese, for garnish

DIRECTIONS

1. Brown beef ovr medium heat in a 6-quart soup pot and drain (rinse in hot water, drain, and return to pot, if desired).

2. Add onion and garlic. Cook until onion is tender.
3. Add remaining Ingredients (except cheese) and bring to a boil over medium-high heat. Reduce heat and simmer for 30 minutes.
4.Taste and adjust seasonings if needed.
5.Serve with Parmesan cheese sprinkled on top, if desired.

Crepes With Ricotta Cocoa Filling

INGREDIENTS

Filling mix

1/4 cup part-skim ricotta cheese
1 dash ground cinnamon
1 g sugar substitute
1/8-1/4 teaspoon cocoa powder

Crepe Mix

2 eggs
2 tablespoons part-skim ricotta cheese
1/2 teaspoon ground cinnamon or 1 dash nutmeg

1 1/2 teaspoons vanilla extract
1 (1 g) packet sugar substitute

DIRECTIONS

1. For the crepe mix, beat the eggs in a small mixing bowl and add the remaining ingredients and beat until well blended.
2. Spray a small skillet, crepe or omelette pan with non stick cooking spray.
3. Pour the crepe mixture into skillet/pan and cook on medium heat until almost cooked through.
4. Meanwhile, combine together the crepe filling ingredients.
5. Flip crepe and cook just a bit more; put filling mixture in a line down the middle and roll crepe over top and cook until done.
6. *You can also flip this like a pancake and top it with the ricotta filling, rather than rolling it over.
7. *Top with sprinkled ground cinnamon, sugar free syrup or a squirt of Redi Whip, optional.

Peanut Butter Muffins

INGREDIENTS

1/2 cup egg white
1/4 cup ground flax seeds
1/4 cup ground almonds
1/4 cup Splenda granular, sugar substitute
1/2 cup natural-style peanut butter
1/4 cup ricotta cheese
1 teaspoon vanilla
1 teaspoon baking soda

DIRECTIONS

1. Preheat oven to 350°F.
2. Melt peanut butter in microwave for 1 minute or until smooth.
3. Mix all ingredients together.
4. Pour into mini muffin cups (24 cup tray), and bake 15 minutes.

Muffin

INGREDIENTS

1 large egg
1 1/2 teaspoons Splenda sugar substitute
1 teaspoon cinnamon (I use more)
2 teaspoons plain fat-free yogurt
1/2 teaspoon baking powder
3 tablespoons ground flax seeds

DIRECTIONS

1. Spray a microwave safe ramekin or bowl with cooking spray (or use a muffin liner).
2. Mix the egg and splenda until well combined (I use a fork), add the yogurt and blend well.
3. Mix in the ground flaxseed, cinnamon and baking powder until well combined.
4. Pour in ramekin and microwave on high for 1 minute 30 seconds (note the ramekin should be no more than half full since these do rise a lot, if it is too small they will overflow).
5. These taste best served hot.

Chocolate Meringue Cookies

INGREDIENTS

3 egg whites
1/8 teaspoon cream of tartar
1/2 teaspoon vanilla extract
2/3 cup Splenda granular (I used a little less than 2/3)
1 tablespoon unsweetened cocoa powder
1 handful of crushed almonds (optional) or 1 pecans (optional)

DIRECTIONS

1. Preheat oven to 300 degrees F (150 degrees C).
2. Combine egg whites, cream of tartar, and vanilla. Beat until the whites form soft peaks. Slowly add sugar substitute and cocoa; beat until stiff peaks form, and mixture becomes glossy.
3. Optional - Fold in nuts.
4. Drop mixture by teaspoonfuls on to a greased cookie sheet. Bake for 25 to 30 minutes.
5. Cool completely and store in an airtight container.

Chocolate Meringue Cookies

INGREDIENTS

3 egg whites
1/8 teaspoon cream of tartar
1/2 teaspoon vanilla extract
2/3 cup Splenda granular (I used a little less than 2/3)
1 tablespoon unsweetened cocoa powder
1 handful of crushed almonds (optional) or 1 pecans (optional)

DIRECTIONS

1. Preheat oven to 300 degrees F (150 degrees C).
2. Combine egg whites, cream of tartar, and vanilla. Beat until the whites form soft peaks. Slowly add sugar substitute and cocoa; beat until stiff peaks form, and mixture becomes glossy.
3. Optional - Fold in nuts.
4. Drop mixture by teaspoonfuls on to a greased cookie sheet. Bake for 25 to 30 minutes.
5. Cool completely and store in an airtight container.

Lettuce Wrap

INGREDIENTS

1 leaf red leaf lettuce or 1 leaf green leaf lettuce
1 slice turkey breast
1 slice ham
1 slice tomatoes
1 slice avocado
1 teaspoon lime juice
1 leaf arugula or 1 leaf watercress
1 tablespoon sugar-free ranch dressing

DIRECTIONS

1. Place lettuce leaf on a plate;.
2. Top with turkey, ham, and tomato.
3. in a small bowl, mash avocado and lime juice, and spread onto the tomato.
4. Top with arugula or watercress and dressing.
5. Roll up and secure with a wooden pick.

Cauliflower - Spinach

INGREDIENTS

1 head cauliflower
1 (10 ounce) bag spinach
1 tablespoon olive oil (more, if needed)
1 teaspoon pre-minced garlic (jarred)
salt and pepper, to taste
Splenda sugar substitute, to taste
red pepper flakes, to taste (optional)

DIRECTIONS

1. Break cauliflower into bite-size florets.
2. Saute in olive oil, adding more oil when (and if) necessary, till cauliflower begins to brown.
3. Add the garlic (more if you like).
4. Stir to combine flavors.
5. Season with salt, pepper, Splenda and red pepper flakes (if desired).
6. Optional: Spinach can be added if desired. Place the fresh spinach on top of the cauliflower once it is browned to you liking. When spinach is wilted, stir to combine. Or, cook spinach separately and add to browned cauliflower, and combine.

Oven Roasted Vegetables

INGREDIENTS

1 medium zucchini
1 medium summer squash
1 medium red bell pepper
1 medium yellow bell pepper
1 lb fresh asparagus
1 red onion, chopped
3 tablespoons extra virgin olive oil
1 teaspoon salt
1/2 teaspoon black pepper

DIRECTIONS

1. Preheat oven to 450 degrees.
2. Cut zucchini, summer squash, red pepper, yellow pepper and asparagus into bite-size pieces.
3. Put all vegetables in a large roasting pan, and toss with the oil, salt and black pepper.
4. Spread in a single layer.
5. Roast for 30 minutes, stirring occasionally, until vegetables are lightly browned and tender.

Chicken and Lentil Stew

INGREDIENTS

1 tablespoon extra virgin olive oil
1 small onion, finely chopped
2 garlic cloves, minced
1/4 teaspoon dried basil
1/4 teaspoon dried oregano
1/8 teaspoon fresh ground black pepper
salt
1 tablespoon tomato paste
1 lb boneless skinless chicken breast, cut crosswise into 1/2 in. slices
15 ounces lentils, can drained and rinsed
14 1/2 ounces diced tomatoes, with juices
3/4 cup low sodium chicken broth
4 ounces Baby Spinach (4 cups)

DIRECTIONS

1. In a medium saucepan, heat oil over medium heat. Add onion, garlic, basil, oregano, pepper, and a pinch

of salt; reduce heat to medium-low and cook, stiring occasionally, 4 minutes.

2. Stir in tomato paste and cook 3 minutes longer.

3. Stir in chicken breasts and cook for 1 minute. Add lentils, tomatoes, and their juices, and broth. Bring to a gentle simmer, reduce heat to low, cover and cook until chicken is cooked through, 7 to 10 minutes.

4. Stir in spinach, cover, and cook 1 minute longer or until spinach wilts. Season with salt and pepper to taste and serve warm.

Sausage Veggie Muffins

INGREDIENTS

1 -2 lb Italian sausage
2 green peppers
1 small onion
4 large eggs

1/2 cup parmesan cheese

DIRECTIONS

1. NOTE: You can use egg substitute (I always keep a container handy).
2. Heat oven to 350.
3. Crumble your italian sauge in a skillet with NO oil until nicely browned. (you can also use the italian patties).
4. Drain on paper towels and set aside in bowl.
5. Chop your peppers and onion and saute in same skillet until soft. Add to your sausages and mix well.
6. Spray your muffin tins and fill 1/2 way with sausage mix. If using whole eggs, beat and pour just to barely cover mix in tins. If using egg substitute, just pour to just barely cover.

7.Sprinkle Parm cheese over top, this will form a nice crust. Place muffin tin on top of large cookie sheet incase of dripping.
8.Bake for 10 - 15 minuters until slightly puffed.
9.There's no seasoning to add because the sausage is pre-seasoned. You can also make this with Turkey Sausage and use whatever veggies you like!

Diet Soup

INGREDIENTS

5 medium carrots, cut into 1 inch slices
3 medium celery ribs, sliced
3 large onions, chopped or 3 medium leeks, each cut into 1 inch slices
1 garlic clove, minced
1 (28 ounce) can tomatoes (in juice)
1/2 medium cauliflower, cut into bite sized pieces
12 ounces green beans, each cut into thirds
3 medium zucchini, cut into 1 inch slices
2 (5 ounce) packages baby spinach leaves
1/2 cup chopped fresh parsley
2 chicken bouillon cubes
12 cups water
1 teaspoon salt
1/2 teaspoon fresh ground pepper

DIRECTIONS

1. Coat pan with nonstick cooking spray.
2. Over medium high heat add carrots, celery, onions,

and garlic.

3. Cook, stirring occasionally, 5 minutes.
4. Stir in tomatoes with their liquid, breaking up tomatoes with side of spoon.
5. Add cauliflower, remaining ingredients and 12 cups of water.
6. Heat to boiling over high heat, stirring occasionally.
7. Reduce heat to low, cover and simmer, stirring occasionally, 15 minutes or until vegetables become tender.
8. Add more salt and pepper if desired.

Steak Diane

INGREDIENTS

4 (3 ounce) beef tenderloin, about
5 tablespoons trans free margarine, i use smart balance
1/4 cup onion, minced
1/4 cup mushroom, sliced
1/2 teaspoon garlic, minced
1 tablespoon Worcestershire sauce
1 teaspoon mustard powder
2 tablespoons lemon juice
1 tablespoon dried parsley

fresh chives (to garnish) (optional)
salt
pepper

DIRECTIONS

1. Place each 3 oz piece of tenderloin between wax paper and pound with a mallet until the steak is about 1/2 inch thick.
2. Pat meat with paper towel to dry; season with salt and pepper.
3. In a large skillet, melt 3 Tbsp of the margarine and cook meat on medium to high heat for 2 minutes on

each side.
4. Remove the meat from skillet onto a plate and keep warm.
5. In the same skillet, melt 2 Tbsp of margarine and saute the mushrooms, onion and garlic until veggies are semi-soft.
6. Add the mustard powder and Worcestershire, mixing well.
7. Add the meat to skillet and cook until meat is done to your liking.
8. Remove the meat and keep warm; combine lemon juice and parsley in the skillet and cook until warmed.
9. Pour sauce over the meat and garnish with chives; serve.

Spaghetti Squash

INGREDIENTS

1 spaghetti squash (mine weighed three pounds when whole before cooking)
1 lb ground turkey breast
3 garlic cloves, minced
1/2 large onion, diced
1 green bell pepper, chopped
28 ounces diced tomatoes
salt and pepper
1 teaspoon italian seasoning
1 cup reduced-fat feta cheese

DIRECTIONS

1. Pierce the squash in several places, put on a plate and microwave until tender (mine took about 20 minutes).
2. Allow cool while you cook the meat and veggie mixture.
3. Brown meat with garlic, onion, salt and pepper, and bell pepper.

4. Drain and add Italian spice and tomatoes.
5. If it seems really liquidy, cook some of the liquid off.
6. Cut the squash in half and scrape out the seeds and discard them.
7. Use a fork to scrape the spaghetti into strands and mix gently with sauce mix.
8. Transfer to a large casserole dish that has been sprayed with cooking spray.
9. Bake uncovered for 35 minutes at 350 degrees.
10. Sprinkle the cheese on top and bake 10-15 minutes more.

Stuffed Bell Peppers

INGREDIENTS

4 bell peppers
olive oil
1 lb ground turkey
1 stalk celery, chopped with top
1 -2 garlic clove, minced
1 small onion, chopped
1 tablespoon minced fresh parsley
1 tablespoon Worcestershire sauce
1 teaspoon spike seasoning (for zest)

28 ounces ground peeled tomatoes
1/2 cup shredded cheese (or more)
salt and pepper

DIRECTIONS

1.Wash the peppers, cut the tops off, and place in oiled glass dish.
2.Cover and microwave the peppers for 5 minutes.
3.Saute the veggies and ground turkey with a dollop of olive oil. (I chop up the usable remainders of the pepper tops as well).

4.Add the tomatoes and seasonings. Cook for 3-4 minutes to evaporate some of the liquid.
5.Stuff the peppers and top with cheese.
6.Bake at 350 for 10 minutes or until the peppers are soft and the cheese is toasted.
7.Add Ins: you could add cooked rice or stir in extra cheese to the mixture before baking.

7 - Day - Soup

INGREDIENTS

3 cups crushed plum tomatoes
2 1/2 cups pasta sauce
1/2 cup tomato paste (1 small can)
6 green onions
2 cups beef broth
1 bunch celery & tops
2 cups fresh green beans
2 green bell peppers
2 lbs carrots
2 teaspoons chili powder
1 teaspoon coarse salt
2 teaspoons paprika
1/8 teaspoon cayenne pepper
2 teaspoons prepared mustard
1 teaspoon ground black pepper

DIRECTIONS

1. In a very large stock pot, combine tomatoes, pasta sauce, tomato paste and beef broth.
2. Over med/high heat, bring mixture to a boil.
3. Reduce heat and simmer covered for 15 minutes.

4. Wash and rough chop carrots, celery (including tops), and green peppers into 1 inch cubes.
5. Wash, trim and cut green beans into 1 inch lengths.
6. Chop green onion into 1/4 inch lengths.
7. Add all vegetables to simmering pot.
8. Stir to combine.

9. Add chili powder, cayenne, mustard, salt, black pepper and paprika to soup mixture.
10. Stir and simmer on low for 60 - 90 minutes.

Soup Diet - Day #1.

Eat as much of any fruit you want EXCEPT BANANAS. Eat only soup and fruit today but eat all you want.

Day #2.

All Veggies.

Fill up on fresh vegetables (salads etc).

Eat all the soup you want and have a large baked potato with butter at dinner time.

But NO FRUIT TODAY.

Day #3.

Eat all the soup, fruit and veggies you want, but NO POTATOES.

If you haven't cheated you will have lost.

5-7 lbs by tomorrow morning.

Day #4.

Bananas and skim milk.

Eat at least 3 bananas and all the milk you want today.

Remember, you can have soup anytime you want.

Day #5.

Beef and Tomatoes.

You can have up to 20 ounces of beef and 6 tomatoes in any style you like.

Remember to eat soup too.

Day #6.

Beef and Vegetables.

Eat all the beef and veggies you want today.

You can have 2-3 steaks if you want, with green leafy vegetables.

But NO POTATOES.

Don't forget to have soup.

Day #7.

Brown rice, unsweetened fruit juice, and veggies today.

Eat all you want whenever you want and have soup as often as you can.
The soup is the key --
If you haven't cheated, you should have lost 10 - 17 lbs.
Prescription medications will not be affected by this diet, but check with you doctor before you begin the diet just to be sure.
Remember; The more soup you eat, the more weight you will lose.

Tiramisu

INGREDIENTS

6 large egg whites
1/2 teaspoon cream of tartar
1/8 teaspoon sea salt
3/4 teaspoon vanilla extract (divided)
1/3 cup Splenda granular, sugar substitute plus
2 teaspoons Splenda granular
6 tablespoons whole wheat pastry flour
1/2 cup part-skim ricotta cheese
1/2 cup fat-free whipped topping (or light)
1/4 cup decaffeinated espresso (strongly brewed)
1/2 teaspoon unsweetened cocoa powder
mint sprig (for garnish) (optional)

DIRECTIONS

1. Heat oven to 350'F.
2. Lightly spray an 8x8 inch baking pan with cooking spray. I use grape seed oil.
3. Using an electric mixer, in a large bowl beat the egg whites at high speed, with the cream of tartar and salt until stiff peaks form. About 5 minutes.
4. Add 1/2 teaspoons of the vanilla extract and beat to

combine. Add 1/3 cup sugar substitute and beat the mixture to form stiff peaks.

5. Sift 2 tablespoons of the flour over the beaten egg whites and fold gently to incorporate. Repeat twice with remaining flour until all the flour is folded into the egg whites.

6. Pour the batter into your prepared pan and gently smooth the top. Bake turning once half way through the cooking time until the cake is golden and the tester comes out clean. About 20 minutes. Cool completely.

7. In a small bowl combine the ricotta, whipped topping, remaining 2 teaspoons sugar substitute, and remaining 1/4 teaspoon vanilla.

8. Cut the cake in half vertically down the middle to make two 4 by 8 inch pieces. Place the halves on a flat work surface.

9. Drizzle 2 tablespoons espresso onto each half. Spread half of the ricotta mixture onto one of the halves and dust with half of the cocoa powder.

10. Top with the remaining cake half; spread the top with the remaining ricotta mixture and dust with remaining cocoa powder.

11. Using a serrated knife, gently cut cake crosswise into 4 slices and serve with mint leaves for garnish if using.

Salmon With Creamy Lemon Sauce Low Carb

INGREDIENTS
1 tablespoon olive oil
1 garlic clove, minced
1/4 cup lemon juice
2 tablespoons capers
1 teaspoon lemon-pepper seasoning
1/2 cup fat free sour cream
1 1/2 lbs salmon fillets

DIRECTIONS

1. Preheat the oven to 350°F.
2. Coat a baking sheet with cooking spray.
3. Heat the oil in a small saucepan over medium heat.
4. Add the garlic and cook for one minute.
5. Reduce heat to low; stir in the lemon juice, capers and lemon-pepper seasoning and cook for 5 minutes.
6. Add the sour cream and cook for 5 minutes or until heated though.
7. Meanwhile, place the salmon on the prepared baking sheet.
8. Bake for 20 minutes or until the fish is just opaque.
9. Serve with the sauce.

Sugar Free Peanut Butter Delight

INGREDIENTS

1 cup part-skim ricotta cheese
2 tablespoons natural-style peanut butter
1 teaspoon vanilla extract
2 teaspoons sugar substitute

DIRECTIONS

1. Blend.
2. Chill.
3. Serve.

Cauliflower Mash With Chives

INGREDIENTS

1 1/2 lbs cauliflower, cut into large florets (about 8 cups)

3 garlic cloves
2 (14 ounce) cans reduced-sodium chicken broth
salt & freshly ground black pepper, to taste
2 teaspoons fresh chives, chopped
3 -4 ounces fat free cream cheese (optional)

DIRECTIONS

1. Combine cauliflower, garlic cloves, and broth in a large saucepan. If cauliflower is not completely covered by the broth, add water until just covered. Bring to a boil, reduce heat to medium-low, and simmer until cauliflower is tender, about 12 minutes.

2. Reserve 2 Tbsp of the cooking liquid and drain cauliflower (don't dry it, but allow it to drain fairly thoroughly). Transfer cauliflower and garlic to the bowl of a food processor, and process until smooth, pulsing

in one or two tbsp of the reserved broth, if necessary, to moisten mixture. You might want to use fat free cream cheese during this step instead of the broth for extra body and creaminess. Season with salt and pepper to taste. Just before serving, stir in chopped chives. Serve warm.

Pepper Crusted Tenderloin of Beef

INGREDIENTS

2 (1 lb) beef tenderloin steaks
4 tablespoons minced shallots
1 tablespoon fresh rosemary
1 teaspoon minced garlic
2 teaspoons salt
2 tablespoons ground black pepper
2 teaspoons orange zest (optional)
3 tablespoons olive oil (approximate)
1 cup white pearl onion

DIRECTIONS

1. Preheat the oven to 375°F.
2. Bring water to boil in a small saucepan.
3. Immerse the onions in boiling water for about 2 minutes, then shock them with cold water.
4. Cut off the root tip of each onion and squeeze it out of the skin.
5. Heat 2 Tablespoon of the olive oil in a large skillet over medium heat.
6. Add the shallots and saute for 2 minutes or until tender.

7. Rub the beef with olive oil.
8. Combine the pepper, salt, garlic, rosemary and orange zest, if using, and pat the mixture on the beef.
9. Increase the heat to high and sear the beef in the pan on all sides.
10. Add the pearl onions and place the skillet directly in the oven.
11. Roast until a thermometer reads 145 degrees for medium rare.

Chicken-Pistachio Salad

INGREDIENTS

Salad
1/2 cup pistachio nut, shelled and finely ground
3/4 teaspoon salt
1/2 teaspoon black pepper, freshly ground (plus a pinch)
4 boneless skinless chicken breast halves
2 tablespoons extra virgin olive oil
1/2 cup sweet white onion, diced
1 head romaine lettuce

Dressing

1 teaspoon sweet white onion, grated
1 large avocado, pitted and peeled
3 tablespoons extra virgin olive oil
3 tablespoons fresh lime juice
1 tablespoon water

DIRECTIONS

To make the salad:.

1. Preheat the oven to 375. Mix the nuts in a pie plate with 1/2 tsp salt and 1/2 tsp pepper. Press the chicken into the nuts. Heat 1 Tbs of the oil in a skillet and cook the breasts, 2 min per side. Place the breasts in a baking dish and bake for 15 min or til thermometer registers 160 and juices run clear.
2. Heat the remaining Tbs of oil in a nonstick skillet over high heat. Add the diced onion, 1/4 tsp salt, and a pinch of pepper. Cook til the onion is browned.
3. Line 4 serving plates with lettuce. Slice the chicken breasts and arrange 1 breast on top of the lettuce on each place. Serve with the dressing.

To make the dressing:.

4. Puree the onion, avocado, oil, lime juice, and water in a blender.

Thai Shrimp Soup With Lime and Cilantro

INGREDIENTS

1 tablespoon canola oil
3 tablespoons fresh ginger, minced
1 small onion, thinly sliced
5 cups reduced-sodium chicken broth
1/4 teaspoon red pepper flakes
1 head napa cabbage, thinly sliced (about 3 cups)
1 1/2 lbs shrimp, peeled and deveined
2 tablespoons asian fish sauce
2 teaspoons lime zest
1/4 cup lime juice
1/2 cup fresh cilantro, chopped or 1/2 cup chopped scallion

DIRECTIONS

5. Heat oil in a large pot.

6. Add ginger and onion.
7. Cook, stirring frequently for about 3 minutes.
8. Add broth and red pepper flakes and bring to a low boil.
9. Add cabbage and cook for approximately 2 to 3

minutes.
10. Add shrimp, lime zest and lime juice.
11. Cook just until shrimp turns pink.
12. Serve hot sprinkled with cilantro or scallions.

Mashed Potatoes

INGREDIENTS

4 cups cauliflower florets
1 ounce butter-flavored cooking spray
1 fluid ounce fat-free half-and-half
1 pinch salt
1 pinch fresh ground pepper

DIRECTIONS

1. Steam or microwave cauliflower until soft.
2. Puree cauliflower in food processor and add butter spray and half and half to taste.

Cheesy Ham Omelet

INGREDIENTS

2 eggs
2 tablespoons nonfat milk
3 slices thin-sliced smoked lunch meat ham, chopped
1 teaspoon green onion, thinly sliced
1 dash black pepper
1/4 cup shredded reduced-fat cheddar cheese

DIRECTIONS

1. Beat eggs and milk in small bowl with fork until blended. Add ham, onion, and pepper; mix well.
2. Spray an 8-in. nonstick skillet with cooking spray.
3. Pour egg mixture into skillet; cover. Cook on medium heat 6 minutes or until egg mixture is set but top is still moist.
4. Sprinkle cheese evenly onto half of omelet. Using spatula, fold egg mixture over filling; cover.
5. Remove from heat; let stand 1 minute.
6. Cut in half to serve.

Pineapple Juice with Rum

INGREDIENTS

2 ounces pineapple juice
2 ounces Bacardi light rum
1 teaspoon sugar
1/2 cup ice, crushed

DIRECTIONS

1. Pour all of the ingredients into a cocktail shaker.
2. Shake vigorously 10 seconds.
3. Strain into a chilled cocktail glass.

Pie

INGREDIENTS

1 (16 ounce) packagefrozen cauliflower florets
1 tablespoon extra virgin olive oil
1 large onion, chopped
2 garlic cloves, minced
1 lb extra lean ground beef
2 cups shelled frozen edamame, defrosted
1/2 cup reduced-sodium beef broth
2 teaspoons Worcestershire sauce
1/2 teaspoon low-fat sour cream
1 large egg yolk
1/2 cup shredded reduced-fat cheddar cheese

DIRECTIONS

1.Heat the oven to 350. Spray a 2 quart casserole with cooking spray.
2.Bring a medium saucepan of water to boil. Add cauliflower and cook until tender, about 10 minutes. Drain and transfer to a large bowl.
3.Meanwhile, in a large skillet, heat oil over medium heat. Add onion and garlic; cook, stirring occasionally, until translucent, about 5 minutes. Add beef and brown

for 10 minutes, stirring to break up lumps. Add edamame and cook, stirring occasionally, 3 minutes longer. Stir in broth and Worcestershire sauce. Season with pepper and a pinch of salt. Transfer meat mixture to the casserole.

4. With an electric mixer at medium speed, whip the cooked cauliflower with sour cream, egg yolk, and another pinch of salt. Spoon cauliflower evenly over meat. Top with cheese and bake for 20 to 25 minutes, or until golden on top. Serve warm.

Haystacks

INGREDIENTS

1 cup Fiber One cereal
1 (1 1/2 ounce) milk chocolate candy bars
1 tablespoon reduced-fat peanut butter

DIRECTIONS

1. Melt bar and peanut butter in microwave until smooth, at 30-second intervals.
2. Be careful not to burn or overcook.
3. Stir chocolate and peanut butter mixture.
4. Add cereal and gently toss till coated.
5. Drop onto wax paper, making 6 stacks.
6. Refrigerate until chocolate hardens (about 30 minutes).

Cola Chicken

INGREDIENTS

4 chicken breasts
nonstick cooking spray
1 cup ketchup
1 (12 ounce) can diet cola (I hear diet orange soda works well also)

DIRECTIONS

1. Spray your pan with cooking spray.
2. Place chicken breasts in pan.
3. Brown lightly on each side.
4. Mix Ketchup and Diet Cola together.
5. Pour over chicken.
6. Cook for about 45 minutes or until chicken is tender.

Cabbage Soup

INGREDIENTS

1 head cabbage, chopped
6 onions, sliced or chopped
2 green bell peppers, chopped
1 bunch celery, chopped
1 bunch shallots or 1 bunch green onion, sliced
2 chicken bouillon cubes
1 (1 1/4 ounce) envelope onion soup
1/2 cup balsamic vinegar (optional)
48 ounces V8 vegetable juice
2 (28 ounce) cans chopped tomatoes
1 lemon, juice of
pepper
6 garlic cloves, crushed

DIRECTIONS

1. Place all in large stock pot and bring to a boil.
2. Simmer for 1 hour.
3. Refrigerate all leftovers.

Chocolate Peanut Butter Muffins

INGREDIENTS

2 eggs
1/2 cup peanut butter
1/2 cup 2% fat cottage cheese
1 teaspoon vanilla
1 teaspoon baking soda
1 tablespoon cocoa powder
8 -10 g artificial sweetener

DIRECTIONS

1. Preheat oven to 350*. Line a cup cake pan with paper cups.
2. Microwave the peanut butter for 45 seconds to melt.

3. Add everything to a medium sized bowl and mix well.
4. 1 packet of artificial sweetener = 1 gram. Spoon into 9 cup cake cups and bake for 15 minutes.

Chicken Capri

INGREDIENTS

4 tablespoons low-fat ricotta cheese (Part Skim)
1/2 teaspoon dried oregano
1 teaspoon fresh parsley, finely minced
1/4 teaspoon salt
1/4 teaspoon fresh cracked pepper
2 tablespoons parmesan cheese
4 boneless skinless chicken breast halves
1/2 teaspoon garlic powder
2 tablespoons extra virgin olive oil
4 tablespoons crushed tomatoes
4 slices reduced-fat mozzarella cheese

DIRECTIONS

1. In a small bowl mash Ricotta Cheese, Parmesan Cheese, Salt, Pepper, Oregano & Parsley together until well blended.

2. Toss the chicken with the garlic powder and brown in the olive oil in a large skillet over medium heat for 10 minutes per side.

3.When done remove to a shallow casserole dish to cool slightly.
4.Preheat oven to 350 degrees.
5.Spoon 1 Heaping serving spoon of Ricotta mixture onto each chicken breast and top with 1 tablespoons of Crushed Tomatoes.
6.Place one slice of mozzarella cheese on each one and place in the top rack of the oven.
7.Bake for 20 minutes until a meat thermometer registers 170 deg. Fahrenheit

Cheerio's Diet Snack

INGREDIENTS

1 egg white
1 tablespoon chili powder
1/2 teaspoon cumin
1/4 teaspoon garlic powder
1/4 teaspoon salt
1/4 teaspoon ground pepper (or pepper sauce)
3 cups Cheerios toasted oat cereal (Reg. or Multi-grain)
nonstick cooking spray

DIRECTIONS

1. Pre-heat oven to 325°F.
2. Whisk egg white until foamy. Mix in spices. Stir in Cheerios or Chex. Coat a large cookie sheet with vegetable spray, and spread mixture on it. Spray the cereal with a light coating of more vegetable spray. Place in oven and stir every 5 minutes, for a total of 15-20 minutes. Cool completely.

Cream of Broccoli Soup

INGREDIENTS

1 1/2 small head of broccoli (about 3 pounds)
3 tablespoons canola oil
1 1/2 cups leeks, sliced (white part only)
3/4 cup celery, sliced
1 1/2 quarts chicken broth, fat-free
3 cups evaporated skim milk
1/3 cup cornstarch
1 1/2 teaspoons fresh thyme, chopped
ground pepper (to taste)

DIRECTIONS

1. Cut the broccoli into florets and set aside.
2. Trim and discard the tough fibrous skin from the stems, coarsely chop and set aside.
3. In a medium saucepan over medium-low heat, warm the oil.
4. Add leeks and celery and saute for 8 minutes, or until the leeks are soft.
5. Add the broccoli stems and broth. Bring to a boil, then reduce the heat to low, cover and simmer for 15

minutes.

6.Add the broccoli florets and simmer for 10 minutes more.

7.Puree the mixture in a food processor or blender. Return to saucepan.

8.In a small bowl, whisk together 1 cup of evaporated milk with the cornstarch until smooth.

9.Slowly add to the broccoli mixture, stirring constantly over medium heat.

10.Stir in the remaining milk, thyme, and pepper. Cook and stir until thickened and bubbly. Cook and stir 2 minutes more.

Pineapple Muffins

INGREDIENTS

2 cups flour
4 teaspoons baking powder
1/3 cup powdered artificial sweetener or 4 (1 g) packages Sweet 'n Low
1/2 teaspoon salt
4 tablespoons melted margarine
19 ounces crushed pineapple
1 beaten egg

DIRECTIONS

1. Combine flour, baking powder, sweetner and salt.
2. Add melted butter.
3. Add beaten egg and 19 oz tin of crushed pineapple.
4. ingredients will be very thick in texture. Line your muffin pan cups with cupcake papers.
5. Bake 18 minutes at 400°F.

Cucumber Water

INGREDIENTS

1 long English cucumber, washed and cut into 1/4-inch slices
12 cups cold water
3 cups ice
cucumber, sliced (to garnish)

DIRECTIONS

1. Place cucumber slices in a large pitcher. Add water and ice cubes and stir.
2. Pour into glasses filled with ice and enjoy!
3. Garnish each glass with cucumber slices - optional of course!

Snickers

INGREDIENTS

1/2 gallon non-fat vanilla frozen yogurt

1 (1 1/2 ounce) box fat-free sugar-free instant chocolate pudding mix
1/2 cup natural chunky peanut butter
1 (8 ounce) container reduced-calorie whipped topping (Cool Whip)
diet fudge topping (optional) or chocolate fudge topping (optional)

DIRECTIONS

1. Let frozen yogurt sit at room temperature to soften slightly (approx 10 minutes).
2. In a large bowl, combine the frozen yogurt, pudding mix and peanut butter.
3. Fold in whipped topping.
4. Spoon into a 13x9-inch pan.
5. If desired drizzle lightly with the fudge or chocolate topping in an attractive pattern.
6. Freeze until firm about 2 hours.

7.Cut into 16 pieces.

Coleslaw

INGREDIENTS

1/4 cup plain nonfat yogurt
2 tablespoons light mayonnaise
1 tablespoon fresh lemon juice
1 teaspoon grated lemon, rind of
1/2 teaspoon celery seed
4 cups thinly shredded green cabbage (from about ½ large head)
1 large carrot, peeled and coarsely grated
1/4 cup chopped red onion
2 tablespoons chopped fresh parsley

DIRECTIONS

1. Whisk yogurt, mayonnaise, lemon juice, lemon peel, and celery seeds in large bowl to blend.
2. Add remaining ingredients; toss to coat.
3. Season to taste with salt and pepper (Can be made 2 hours ahead).
4. Cover; chill.

5. Toss before serving.

Chicken Piccata

INGREDIENTS

3/4 lb whole skinless boneless chicken breast, halved lengthwise
2 tablespoons dry sherry
1 tablespoon capers
1 tablespoon extra virgin olive oil
2 tablespoons trans-free margarine
1/4 teaspoon paprika
2 tablespoons minced fresh parsley
1 tablespoon lemon juice
salt and pepper

DIRECTIONS

1. Pound the chicken pieces to flatten them slightly. Season them with salt and pepper to taste.
2. Heat an empty pan on high heat, then add the oil and one tablespoon of the margarine and allow that to get

hot (but not smoking). Then carefully add the chicken, making sure the oil doesn't splatter. Doing this process will prevent the chicken from sticking. If you heat the oil and pan together, or if the pan isn't hot enough, the chicken will stick.

3. Sauté the chicken pieces for 1 minute on each side, or until they are cooked through. Transfer the chicken with tongs to a platter and cover it loosely to keep it warm.

4. Pour off any remaining fat and oil from the skillet.

5. Return it to the stovetop and add the remaining 1 tablespoon margarine, the sherry, and the lemon juice, and bring the mixture to a boil.

6. Stir in the capers, the parsley, the paprika, and salt and pepper to taste, and spoon the sauce over the chicken.

Wasabi-Ginger Glazed Tuna Steaks

INGREDIENTS

2 tablespoons low sodium soy sauce, divided
4 (6 ounce) tuna steaks (1 inch thick)
2 tablespoons ginger marmalade (substitute dried, fresh or pressed pickled ginger for healthier)
2 teaspoons wasabi paste
cooking spray
2 tablespoons fresh cilantro, chopped

DIRECTIONS

1. Spoon 1 tablespoon soy sauce over fish and let stand 5 minutes.
2. Combine the remaining 1 tablespoon soy sauce, ginger, and 2 teaspoons wasabi paste in a small bowl, stirring with a whisk.
3. Heat a grill pan over medium-high heat.
4. Coat pan with cooking spray. Add fish to pan; cook 2 minutes on each side.
5. Spoon marmalade mixture over tuna.
6. Cook 1 minute or to desired wellness (recommend rare as best, medium-rare at maximum).

7. Remove tuna from pan.
8. Sprinkle with cilantro.

Tomato Salad

INGREDIENTS

1 cup seeded, finely diced cucumber
1 teaspoon salt
1 cup finely diced tomato
1 cup finely diced sweet onion (such as Vidalia®)
1 cup finely chopped fresh parsley

3/4 cup finely chopped mint, or to taste
2 tablespoons olive oil, or more to taste
1 tablespoon fresh lemon juice, or more to taste
salt and ground black pepper to taste

DIRECTIONS

1. Place diced cucumber into a colander and sprinkle with 1 teaspoon salt or as needed; allow to drain for about 15 minutes.
2. Toss drained cucumber with tomato, sweet onion, parsley, and mint.
3. Drizzle salad with olive oil and fresh lemon juice and season with salt and black pepper.

4. Serve immediately.

Mexican Soup

INGREDIENTS

4 (6 ounce) skinless, boneless chicken breast halves
1 (28 ounce) can whole peeled tomatoes, drained
1 (10 ounce) can diced tomatoes with green chile peppers
2 tablespoons olive oil
1 medium onion, chopped
1 tablespoon chopped fresh garlic
1 (32 fluid ounce) container chicken broth
1 (14.5 ounce) can kidney beans, rinsed and drained
1 (14.5 ounce) can black beans, rinsed and drained
cayenne pepper to taste
chili powder to taste
Cheddar cheese, shredded
sour cream, for topping

DIRECTIONS

1.Preheat the oven broiler.
2.Arrange chicken breasts in a large pan, and broil 15 minutes in the preheated oven. Remove chicken, allow to cool, then shred.
3.In a food processor or blender, puree the drained

whole tomatoes and diced tomatoes.

4.Heat olive oil in a large skillet over medium heat. Stir in onion and garlic; cook until onion is soft and translucent.

5.Stir in chicken broth and pureed tomatoes. Add shredded chicken, kidney beans, and black beans.

6.Season with cayenne pepper and chili powder. Bring to a boil; then cover, leaving the lid slightly ajar, and simmer 2 hours.

7.Ladle into bowls, and top with cheese and dollops of sour cream.

Zucchini Lasagna With Beef and Sausage

INGREDIENTS

1/2 pound ground beef
1/2 pound bulk Italian sausage
1 onion, chopped
4 cloves garlic, minced
2 tablespoons chopped fresh basil
2 tablespoons chopped fresh oregano
2 tablespoons brown sugar
1 tablespoon red pepper flakes, or to taste
1 teaspoon salt
1/2 teaspoon ground black pepper
1 (14.5 ounce) can diced tomatoes
1 (12 ounce) can tomato paste
2 eggs
2 cups ricotta cheese
1 cup grated Parmesan cheese
1 tablespoon chopped fresh parsley

1 teaspoon salt
3 large zucchini, trimmed
2 cups shredded mozzarella cheese, divided
2 tablespoons grated Parmesan cheese

1 cup shredded mozzarella cheese

DIRECTIONS

1. Cook and stir ground beef, Italian sausage, onion, and garlic in a large skillet over medium heat until the meat is crumbly and no longer pink, about 10 minutes.
2. Drain grease and stir basil, oregano, brown sugar, red pepper flakes, 1 teaspoon salt, black pepper, tomatoes, and tomato paste into the meat. Bring to a boil, reduce heat to low, and simmer meat sauce for 30 minutes. Stir occasionally.
3. Preheat oven to 375 degrees F (190 degrees C). Grease a 9x13-inch baking dish.
4. Mix eggs, ricotta cheese, 1 cup Parmesan cheese, parsley, and 1 teaspoon salt in a bowl until thoroughly combined.
5. Pare several slices of skin lengthwise from zucchini, alternating with strips of remaining skin. Cut zucchini into long strips to resemble lasagna noodles. Discard seedy middle strips.
6. Place 1/3 of the zucchini strips into bottom of the prepared baking dish, filling in any gaps with scrap pieces of zucchini.
7. Spread half the ricotta mixture over zucchini; spread 1 cup of mozzarella cheese over ricotta mixture; spread 1/3 of the meat sauce over mozzarella cheese.
8. Repeat layers once more, layering 1/3 of zucchini

strips, remaining half of the ricotta mixture, 1 more cup of mozzarella cheese, and 1/3 of the meat sauce.

9. Make a third layer of remaining zucchini strips, remaining meat sauce, and 2 tablespoons Parmesan cheese sprinkled on top.

10. Bake in the preheated oven until lasagna is bubbling and top is browned, about 1 hour. If top is browning too quickly, cover dish with aluminum foil during last 15 minutes of baking time.

11. Spread 1 cup mozzarella cheese on top of the casserole and bake until mozzarella cheese topping is melted, 5 to 10 more minutes.

12. Let casserole stand 10 minutes before serving.

Blueberry Ginger Mojito Pitchers

- All out: 40 min
- Prep: 20 min
- Latent: 15 min
- Cook: 5 min
- **Yield: 2 servings**

Fixings

For the Ginger basic syrup:

1/4 cup ground crisp ginger

1 cup granulated sugar

1 cup cold water

For the Mojito:

1 cup crisp blueberries

1 lime, cut into wedges

20 to 24 crisp mint leaves

4 ounces ginger basic syrup

4 ounces vodka

5 ounces club pop

Ice solid shapes

Blueberries, for topping

Mint leaves, for topping
Headings

1.Strip and mesh the ginger and include it, together with the sugar and cold water, to a pot. Carry it to the bubble and mix until the sugar breaks up. Spread and let soak for 15 minutes. Strain and cool in the icebox when done.

2.Include the blueberries, lime wedges and crisp mint leaves to the glass (or pitcher). Obfuscate with a wooden spoon so the blueberries are broken and the mint and lime discharge their juices and flavor. On the off chance that gathering pitchers you can cover them at this stage and leave in the fridge until prepared to serve.

3.At the point when prepared to serve, include the basic syrup, vodka and top off with club pop. Give it a brisk blend and afterward fill glasses with ice 3D shapes. Enhancement with a bunch of crisp blueberries and a sprig of mint.

4.Join the blueberries, mint leaves and lime wedges in the pitcher and jumble it in there with the back of a wooden spoon. When you are prepared to serve include the vodka, ginger basic syrup and club pop. Mix and fill glasses with several ice solid shapes. Topping each glass with some crisp blueberries and a sprig of new mint.

Wavy Endive, Prosciutto and Mozzarella on Bruschetta

- All out: 35 min
- Prep: 20 min
- Cook: 15 min
- **Yield: 6 servings**

Fixings

18 askew cuts (1/2-inch-thick) roll bread

3 tablespoons extra-virgin olive oil

1 head of wavy endive or frisee leaves, isolated into 2-inch strips

1 (7-ounce) ball new water-stuffed mozzarella cheddar, depleted, cut into 18 slim cuts

18 paper-slim cuts prosciutto

2 tablespoons Red Wine Vinaigrette, formula pursues

Red Wine Vinaigrette:

1/2 cup red wine vinegar

1/4 cup new lemon juice

2 teaspoons nectar

2 teaspoons salt

3/4 teaspoon newly ground dark pepper

1 cup extra-virgin olive oil
Bearings

1.Preheat the stove to 350 degrees F.

2.Orchestrate the bread cuts on 2 overwhelming huge heating sheets. Brush 3 tablespoons of oil over the bread cuts. Prepare until the crostini are pale brilliant and fresh, around 15 minutes.

3.Wrap 1 wavy endive and 1 cut of cheddar with 1 cut of prosciutto, enabling the tops to expand 1-inch more than 1 long side of the prosciutto. Organize the crostini on a platter. Top every crostini with a prosciutto roll. Sprinkle the vinaigrette over and serve.

Red Wine Vinaigrette:

1.Blend the vinegar, lemon juice, nectar, salt, and pepper in a blender. With the machine running, bit by bit mix in the oil. Season the vinaigrette, to taste, with progressively salt and pepper, whenever wanted.

Astounding Fried Chicken

- All out: 40 min
- Prep: 10 min
- Latent: 15 min
- Cook: 15 min
- Yield: 4 to 6 servings

Fixings

Canola oil, for singing

2 tablespoons granulated garlic

2 tablespoons granulated onion

2 tablespoons fit salt, in addition to extra for flavoring

2 tablespoons naturally ground dark pepper

1 tablespoon cayenne

1 tablespoon paprika

2 (3 1/2-pound) entire chickens, cut into 10 pieces each and cut back of excess

4 cups universally handy flour

Headings

1.In an enormous skillet, include canola oil over medium warmth.

2.In a little bowl, combine all flavors. Utilize 1/2 of blend to season chicken. Let prepared chicken sit at room temperature for 15 minutes.

3.In a huge bowl, include flour and remaining flavoring blend. Hurl chicken with prepared flour and add to hot oil, 1 piece at once. Spread container with foil. Expel foil following 8 to 10 minutes and flip chicken. Cook until the chicken is brilliant dark colored. Expel from fryer to a paper towel-lined sheet plate. Season with salt, whenever wanted, and serve.

Smoked Salmon Spread

- Absolute: 25 min
- Prep: 25 min
- Yield: 1/2 pints

Fixings

8 ounces cream cheddar, at room temperature

1/2 cup acrid cream

1 tablespoon crisply crushed lemon juice

1 tablespoon minced crisp dill

1 teaspoon arranged horseradish, depleted

1/2 teaspoon fit salt

1/4 teaspoon naturally ground dark pepper

1/4 pound (4 ounces) smoked salmon, minced

Headings

1.Cream the cheddar in an electric blender fitted with an oar connection until simply smooth. Include the harsh cream, lemon juice, dill, horseradish, salt, and pepper, and blend. Include the smoked salmon and blend well. Chill and present with crudites or wafers.

2.On the off chance that you can discover it, I lean toward Norwegian salmon; it's drier and less salty than other smoked salmon.

Hawaiian Beef Teriyaki

- All out: 8 hr 30 min
- Prep: 20 min
- Inert: 8 hr
- Cook: 10 min
- **Yield: 4 servings**

Fixings

1/2 pounds sirloin steak, cut into 1/4-inch strips

3/4 cup soy sauce

1/2-inch cut new ginger

1 clove garlic, minced

1/2 teaspoons dark colored sugar

1/2 cup water

1 pineapple, stripped and cut longwise

1 tablespoon chiffonade or daintily cut mint leaves

Bearings

1.Consolidate soy sauce, ginger, garlic, sugar and water. Marinate meat in the blend in a plastic pack medium-term in the fridge.

2.Preheat the flame broil to high warm. Stick meat on sticks. Cook over hot coals until done just as you would prefer, around 4 to 5 minutes for medium uncommon.

3.Spot pineapple cuts on flame broil. Cook on the two sides until there are flame broil marks and the regular sugars have helped it to dark colored, around 2 minutes for each side.

4.Spot meat sticks over flame broiled pineapple cuts and topping with mint.

Clam Rocks at the Rib

- All out: 45 min
- Prep: 30 min
- Cook: 15 min
- Yield: 4 to 6 servings

Fixings

2 1/2 pounds crisp steamed spinach, depleted

1 medium onion, minced

1 cup ground Parmesan

4 tablespoons (1/2 stick) margarine, softened

1/4 cup white wine

1/2 teaspoon cayenne pepper

1/2 teaspoon dark pepper

2 dozen crisp crude clams

6 enormous cuts ready red tomato, quartered

6 enormous cuts provolone cheddar, quartered

Lemon wedges, for serving

Hot sauce, for serving

Headings

1. Preheat the broiler to 400 degrees F.

2. In a little bowl join the spinach, onion, Parmesan, margarine, wine, cayenne pepper, and dark pepper. Shuck the shellfish and leave them on the half shell. Top with a storing tablespoon of the spinach blend and mastermind them on a preparing sheet. Heat for around 10 minutes. Expel from the broiler and top each with a cut of tomato and cheddar. Come back to the broiler and prepare until the cheddar softens.

3. Move the clams to a serving platter and present with a wedge of lemon and great hot sauce. Appreciate!

Cook's Note

The hardest piece of this formula is to discover new shellfish and shuck them.

Manhattan

- Complete: 5 min
- Prep: 5 min
- Yield: 4 servings

Fixings

6 ice 3D squares

1/4 cup sweet vermouth

1 cup whiskey bourbon

Mixed drink fruits, to enhance

Bearings

1. Put the ice 3D squares in a mixed drink shaker. Pour the vermouth and bourbon over the ice. Shake and after that strain into mixed drink glasses. Include a cherry, whenever wanted, and serve.

Early lunch Breads

- Complete: 1 hr 10 min
- Prep: 20 min
- Inert: 15 min
- Cook: 35 min
- **Yield: 6 to 8 servings for each portion**

Fixings

Essential Bread Mix:

3 (1/4 ounce/7 gram) sachets dried yeast

pounds (1 kilogram) bread flour, in addition to additional flour, for cleaning.

A little more than 1 16 ounces lukewarm water (625 milliliters)

2 level tablespoons ocean salt

1 ounce (30 grams) sugar
Flavorful Rolled Bread of Parma Ham, Egg, Cheese, Egg, and Basil:

10 cuts Parma ham

8 huge natural eggs, bubbled for 8 minutes and shelled

14 ounces (400 grams) cheddar (a blend of Cheddar, Parmesan, Fontina, mozzarella, or any remains that should be spent), ground

2 bunches new basil

Sun-dried tomatoes

Extra-virgin olive oil

Ocean salt and newly ground dark pepper

Hacked new rosemary leaves

Sweet Rolled Bread of Chocolate, Hazelnut, and Banana:

1 container chocolate spread

Hacked toasted hazelnuts

2 bananas, cut
Bearings

1. Essential Bread Mix: Mix every one of the fixings together and work into a mixture. Cut the mixture down the middle.

2. Fold one bit of batter out into a long rectangular shape around 1/2 inch (1 centimeter) thick, around 39 1/2 inches (1 meter) long and 12 to 15 inches wide.

3.Appetizing: Along the center of the principal bit of took off batter, spread out your Parma ham, eggs, cheddar, basil, and tomatoes. Sprinkle with olive oil and season with salt and newly ground dark pepper. Draw the batter over the filling so it structures what resembles a cannelloni shape.

4.Bring one end round to the next with the goal that they sign up. Squeeze and pat the two finishes together immovably to frame a donut formed bread. Brush on olive oil and sprinkle the portion with a little ocean salt and rosemary. Move to a heating plate tidied with flour and permit to confirmation for 15 minutes.

5.Spot in a preheated 400 degrees F (200 degrees C) broiler until brilliant, around 35 minutes.

6.Sweet: On the second bit of the took off batter utilize a palette blade to cover the surface with chocolate spread. Sprinkle some toasted slashed hazelnuts and the cut banana onto the batter. Fold up into a cannelloni shape and afterward roll the long snake shape inside itself to frame a snail shape. Sprinkle with hacked hazelnuts. Move to a heating plate cleaned with flour and permit to verification for 15 minutes.

7.Prepare in a preheated 400 degrees F (200 degrees C) for 35 minutes.

Chocolate Chip Walnut Cupcakes

- Complete: 1 hr 15 min
- Prep: 10 min
- Inert: 40 min
- Cook: 25 min
- **Yield: 12 cupcakes**

Fixings

Cupcakes:
1/2 cup finely cleaved pecans

1 cup smaller than normal semisweet chocolate chips, in addition to 1/4 cup for enhancement

1 (21-ounce) box brownie blend (suggested: Duncan Hines Chewy Fudge)

2 eggs, at room temperature

1/2 cup vegetable oil

1/4 cup water
Icing:

4 ounces mascarpone cheddar, at room temperature
4 ounces cream cheddar, at room temperature
3 cups powdered sugar, filtered

Bearings

1. Exceptional hardware: 12 paper cupcake liners, a 12-cup biscuit dish

2. For the cupcakes: Place a stove rack in the broiler. Preheat the stove to 350 degrees F. Line a 12-cup biscuit container with paper liners.

3. In a little bowl join the pecans, 1 cup smaller than expected chocolate chips and 1 tablespoon of the brownie blend. Hurl until every one of the fixings are covered. Put in a safe spot.

4. In an enormous bowl combine the rest of the brownie blend, eggs, vegetable oil, and water. Mix for 20 seconds until mixed. Crease in the pecans and chocolate chips. Spoon the blend into the readied skillet (cupcake liners will be full). Heat for 22 to 25 minutes until a cake analyzer embedded into the cupcakes turns out with wet fudgy morsels. Cool the cupcakes in the search for gold minutes. Move the cupcakes to a wire rack and cool totally before icing, around 30 minutes.

5. For the icing: In a huge bowl, utilizing an electric hand blender, beat the cheeses together until light and fleecy, around 2 minutes. Bit by bit beat in the

powdered sugar until smooth and spreadable. Refrigerate the icing until prepared to utilize.

6.Spread the icing over the cupcakes and enhancement with the staying small scale chocolate chips. Refrigerate until prepared to serve. Serve at room temperature.

Crab and Potato Frittata

- All out: 1 hr
- Dynamic: 5 min
- **Yield: 6 to 8 servings**

Fixings

1 enormous Yukon gold potato

Genuine salt

6 enormous eggs

1/2 cup creamer

1 teaspoon ground lemon pizzazz

1/2 teaspoon smoked paprika

1 teaspoon olive oil

1 cup kind sized protuberance crabmeat

1/2 cup infant arugula, hacked

Headings

1. Put the potato in a pot with enough water to cover. Season the water liberally with salt and spot over high heat. Heat to the point of boiling and stew for 10 minutes. Channel well and let cool marginally. Cut into quarters and cut into dainty pieces.

2. Preheat the stove to 375 degrees F.

3. In a medium bowl, whisk together the eggs, cream, lemon pizzazz, paprika and 1 teaspoon salt.

4. Oil a 8-inch square preparing dish with the olive oil. In the heating dish, consolidate the crab, arugula and cut potatoes, ensuring the potatoes are altogether lying level. Pour the egg blend over the top.

5. Prepare until the inside is simply set and the top is dark colored, around 30 minutes. Permit to cool for 10 minutes before cutting into 1-inch squares.

Long Island Iced Tea

- All out: 10 min
- Prep: 5 min
- Cook: 5 min
- **Yield: 1 serving**

Fixings

6 ice solid shapes

1/2 jigger gin

1/2 jigger vodka

1/2 jigger white rum

1/2 jigger tequila

1/2 jigger Cointreau

1 jigger crisp lemon juice

1/2 teaspoon sugar syrup (see note)

Cola

Lemon cut, to enhance

Headings

1. Put the ice solid shapes in a blending glass. Include the gin, vodka, rum, tequila, Cointreau, lemon squeeze and sugar syrup. Mix well, at that point strain into a tall glass loaded up with ice 3D shapes. Add enough Coca Cola to fill the glass, and finish with the cut of lemon.

Cook's Note

2. To make sugar syrup, heat 1 cup sugar and 1 cup water in a little pot until the sugar breaks down.

Flame broiled Corn on the Cob with BBQ Butter

- Complete: 1 hr 15 min
- Prep: 10 min
- Inert: 40 min
- Cook: 25 min
- **Yield: 4 servings**

Fixings

2 tablespoons canola oil

1/2 little red onion, hacked

2 cloves garlic, hacked

1 tablespoon ancho stew powder

2 teaspoons Spanish paprika

1 teaspoon toasted cumin seeds

1/2 teaspoon cayenne powder

1/2 cup water

1/2 sticks unsalted spread, somewhat mollified

1 teaspoon Worcestershire sauce

Salt and newly ground dark pepper

Consummately Grilled Corn:

4 ears corn

Legitimate salt
Bearings

1. Consummately Grilled Corn, formula pursues

2. Warmth the oil in a medium saute dish over high heat until practically smoking. Include the onion and cook until delicate, 2 to 3 minutes. Include the garlic and cook for 30 seconds. Include the ancho powder, paprika, cumin and cayenne and cook for 1 moment.

Include 1/2 cup of water and cook until the blend winds up thickened and the water diminishes. Let cool marginally.

3.Spot the spread in a nourishment processor, include the zest blend and Worcestershire sauce and procedure until smooth. Season with salt and pepper, scratch the blend into a little bowl, spread and refrigerate for at any rate 30 minutes to enable the flavors to merge. Bring to room temperature before serving and spread the margarine over the corn while hot.

Flawlessly Grilled Corn:

1.Warmth the flame broil to medium.

2.Force the external husks down the ear to the base. Strip away the silk from every ear of corn by hand. Overlap husks once again into the right spot and tie the closures together with kitchen string. Spot the ears of corn in a huge bowl of virus water with 1 tablespoon of salt for 10 minutes.

3.Expel corn from water and shake off overabundance. Spot the corn on the flame broil, close the spread and barbecue for 15 to 20 minutes, turning at regular intervals, or until bits are delicate when punctured with a paring blade. Evacuate the husks and eat on the cob or expel the bits.

4.The most effective method to expel corn parts from cob: To expel pieces from cobs of either crude or cooked corn, stand cob upstanding on its stem end in a huge container, holding tip with fingers. Chop down the sides of cob with sharp paring blade, discharging portions without cutting into cob. Run dull edge of blade down the cob to discharge any outstanding corn and fluid.

5.Yield: 4 servings

Spaghetti with Summer Squash and Tomatoes

- Complete: 35 min
- Prep: 15 min
- Cook: 20 min
- **Yield: 4 servings**

Fixings

Legitimate salt

1 zucchini, cut into slim rounds

1 summer squash, cut into flimsy rounds

1 16 ounces cherry tomatoes

1/2 onion, finely hacked

1 garlic clove, hacked

1 tablespoon hacked crisp oregano leaves

1/4 cup extra-virgin olive oil

Newly ground dark pepper

1 pound spaghetti

Bearings

1. Heat a huge pot of salted water to the point of boiling over high heat for the spaghetti.

2. Preheat the broiler to 400 degrees F.

3. Join the squashes, tomatoes, onion, garlic, and oregano in a huge bowl. Include the olive oil, sprinkle with salt and pepper, and give it every one of the a decent hurl. Dump that out onto a preparing sheet and meal for 10 to 12 minutes, until the squash is delicate and caramelized. Scratch the vegetables into a huge pasta bowl and spread with a plate to keep everything warm.

4. The pasta water ought to bubble at this point. Add the spaghetti and mix to isolate the strands. Cook for 8 to 9 minutes, until still somewhat firm.

5. To complete, scoop out around 1/4 cup of the pasta cooking water, channel the pasta, and hurl tenderly

with the broiled vegetables and Grilled Shrimp. Include the pasta water if necessary.

Flame broiled Kale Salad with Roasted Sungolds

Complete: 35 min

Dynamic: 20 min

Yield: 4 servings

Fixings

1/2 cup newly ground Parmesan

2 tablespoons lemon juice

Olive oil

Legitimate salt

1 cup split Sungold tomatoes

1/4 teaspoon red pepper chips

1 pack wavy kale, stems expelled

1 little pack Tuscan kale, stems expelled, finely cleaved

1 avocado, diced

1/4 cup cut almonds, toasted

Bearings

1. Whisk together the Parmesan, lemon juice, 3 tablespoons olive oil and 1/2 teaspoon salt in a medium bowl. Put in a safe spot.

2. Preheat the stove to 375 degrees F. Warmth a flame broil or barbecue skillet to high.

3. On a rimmed preparing sheet, hurl the tomatoes with 1 tablespoon olive oil, 1/3 teaspoon salt and the red pepper chips. Move to the broiler and meal until brilliant dark colored and wrinkled, around 30 minutes. Let cool.

4. In the mean time, place the wavy kale leaves legitimately on the hot flame broil. Flame broil for around 1 moment for every side, until withered and singed. Evacuate to a cutting board, cleave into reduced down pieces and add to the bowl with the dressing. Include the crude Tuscan kale, avocado, almonds and tomatoes to the bowl; hurl to coat.

Peaches in Sauternes

- Absolute: 24 min
- Prep: 20 min
- Dormant: 2 min

- Cook: 2 min
- **Yield: 4 to 6 servings**

Fixings

6 to 8 exceptionally ready yellow or white peaches
3 tablespoons sugar
1 (375 ml.) bottle great Sauternes
1 tablespoon orange-seasoned alcohol (suggested: Grand Marnier)

Bearings

1.Heat a pot of water to the point of boiling and submerge the peaches in the water for 1 to 2 minutes, until the skins fall off effectively. Expel them with an opened spoon and spot them in a bowl of virus water to stop the cooking. Strip the peaches and after that cut them in wedges off the pit and into a bowl. Mix in the sugar, Sauternes, and orange alcohol. Spread and refrigerate for in any event 2 hours, or medium-term. Serve cool however not cold.

Container Seared Florida Pompano and Spiny Lobster in Squab Consomme, and Poached Foie Gras

- Absolute: 5 hr
- Prep: 1 hr
- Cook: 4 hr
- **Yield: 4 servings**

Fixings

1 tablespoon spread

4 pompano filets, bloodline expelled

Salt and white pepper, for flavoring

Squab Consomme, formula pursues

4 (1-ounce cuts) foie gras

1 cup celeriac, chiffonade

1 little dark truffle, julienned

2 bulbs spring garlic, shaved fine

2 spiked lobster tails, poached until medium uncommon and cut into 1/4-inch emblems Sprigs chervil, for enhancement

Squab Stock:

2 squab, boned, bosom and leg meat held for Squab Consomme, formula pursues (may substitute 1 duck, arranged a similar way)

1 cup stripped and slashed carrot

1 cup stripped and slashed onion

1 cup stripped and slashed celeriac

4 cups chicken stock

15 entire white peppercorns

Sprig thyme

Sprig rosemary

Squab Consomme:

4 squab bosom and leg meat, held from above

4 egg whites, softly beaten

1 stalk crisp lemon grass, cleaved

5 star anise, squashed

1/3 cup sherry vinegar

1 little beet, stripped and slashed

1 cup stripped and slashed carrot

1 cup stripped and slashed onion

1 cup stripped and slashed celeriac

Squab Stock, see formula above

Headings

1.In an enormous saute container or skillet, liquefy the margarine over medium-high heat. Season the pompano with salt and white pepper. Spot the fish, skin-side down, in the skillet and burn for 2 minutes. Turn fish and cook 1 moment longer. Expel from warmth.

2.In a little pan warm roughly 1 cup of Squab Consomme over low heat, yet don't permit to stew. Include the foie gras and cook for around 4 minutes.

3.In the base of four shallow dishes, organize the celeriac chiffonade, dark truffle, spring garlic, and lobster emblems, partitioning equally between the dishes. Top with the foie gras and fish. Pour the hot Squab Consomme over the top. Embellishment with chervil and serve.

Squab Stock:

1.Preheat a medium pan over medium-high heat. Cut the squab remains into little pieces and spot in the pan. Blend incidentally until the bones are dull dark colored. Include the carrots, onion, and celeriac. Cook and blend until the onions are translucent. Include the chicken stock, white peppercorns, thyme and rosemary. Bring to a light stew, lower warmth to medium, and permit to cook for 2 hours.

Channel, cool, and save stock.

Squab Consomme:

1.In a nourishment processor, beat the saved squab bosom and leg meat until fine.

2.In a huge blending bowl, place the squab meat, egg whites, lemon grass, star anise, sherry vinegar, beets, carrots, onion, and celeriac. Blend in the cooled Squab Stock and spot blend in a limited, high-sided stockpot over medium warmth. Mixing always, keep cooking while persistently scratching the base of the pot to abstain from staying. At the point when the pontoon starts to shape, quit mixing and screen the warmth intently. Try not to enable the fluid to bubble. At the point when the consomme starts to stew through the pontoon, keep cooking for roughly 30 minutes.

3.Utilizing a little spoon, tenderly cause an opening in the pontoon where the consomme to can pool, at that point scoop the pooled consomme into a fine strainer fixed with cheesecloth. Put in a safe spot for administration.

Chocolate S'mores

Complete: 11 min

Prep: 10 min

Cook: 1 min

Yield: 1 serving

Fixings

1 marshmallow

2 chocolate stomach related rolls

Bearings

1.String a marshmallow onto a stick or stick and toast it over an open fire. Sandwich the cooked marshmallow between the 2 rolls.

Tzatziki

Complete: 16 hr 5 min

Prep: 8 hr 5 min

Cook: 8 hr

Fixings

2 cups Mediterranean-style yogurt, (may substitute with customary yogurt)

1 huge English cucumber (stripped, destroyed and depleted)

1 clove garlic, hacked fine

1 tablespoon mint, hacked

1 tablespoon dill, cleaved

1 ounces lemon juice

Salt and pepper to taste

Bearings

1.To Prepare the Yogurt: Line strainer with cheesecloth and set over a bowl. Bowl should bolster strainer so it doesn't contact the base of the bowl. Put the yogurt in the strainer approximately secured, and let it channel medium-term in the refrigerator.Discard the fluid and utilize the stressed yogurt as coordinated.

2.Consolidate all fixings and refrigerate medium-term before serving. Present with pita.

Meat and Broccoli Salad

Absolute: 23 min

Prep: 15 min

Cook: 8 min

Yield: 4 servings

Fixings

4 (6-ounce) bits of meat tenderloin steak, 1-inch thick

Salt and pepper

Vegetable oil cooking splash

1 head broccoli, stem cut of fiberous skin, cut in florets and stem cut into pieces

1 sack blended child greens, 6 to 8 ounces

1 red chime pepper, seeded and in all respects meagerly cut

4 scallions, cut on an edge, 1-inch pieces

1 cup pea pods, cut on a point

1 cup destroyed carrots

8 hot cherry peppers or pepperoncini, cleaved

2 tablespoons cleaved cilantro leaves, discretionary

Dressing:

1/4 cup duck sauce or sweet and acrid sauce

1-inch ginger root, finely cleaved

1 lime, squeezed

2 tablespoons rice wine vinegar or white vinegar

1/2 to 1 teaspoon squashed red pepper pieces

1/4 cup vegetable oil

Headings

1.Preheat flame broil container over high heat. Season steak with salt and pepper. Shower barbecue container with cooking splash. Barbecue meat 3 to 5 minutes for each side for medium uncommon to medium well doneness. Evacuate meat and let stand 10 minutes.

2.In a container, carry 1-inch of water to an air pocket. Include a spot of salt and broccoli pieces and steam for 3 to 5 minutes, until cooked yet at the same time firm. In the sink, channel broccoli in colander and run cold water over it to cool.

3.Organize greens on enormous platter or individual supper plates. Mastermind broccoli and veggies on greens. Consolidate duck or sweet and acrid sauce with ginger, lime juice, vinegar, squashed pepper pieces. Speed in oil. Cut steaks and orchestrate on serving of mixed greens and shower finished dish with dressing. Season with extra salt and pepper.

Swordfish and Spaghetti with Citrus Pesto

Absolute: 35 min

Prep: 15 min

Cook: 20 min

Yield: 4 servings

Fixings

For the Citrus pesto:

1 pound spaghetti pasta (suggested: Barilla)

1 pack new basil, around 3 cups leaves

1/2 cup toasted pine nuts

1 clove garlic

1 lemon, get-up-and-go ground and squeezed

1 orange, get-up-and-go ground and squeezed

1/2 teaspoon salt

1/2 teaspoon crisply ground dark pepper

1/2 cup extra-virgin olive oil

1 cup ground Parmesan

For the Swordfish:

4 (6-ounce) swordfish steaks

Extra-virgin olive oil

Salt and crisply ground dark pepper

Bearings

1. Heat a huge pot of salted water to the point of boiling over high heat. Include the pasta and cook until delicate yet at the same time firm to the chomp, mixing once in a while, around 8 to 10 minutes. Channel pasta and save 1/2 cup of the pasta fluid.

2. Mix the basil, pine nuts, garlic, charms, squeezes, salt, and pepper in a nourishment processor until the blend is finely slashed. With the machine running, step by step include the olive oil until the blend is smooth and velvety. Move to a bowl and blend in the Parmesan. Hurl with the warm spaghetti and the held pasta water.

3. In the interim, place a flame broil skillet over medium-high heat or preheat a gas or charcoal barbecue. Brush the two sides of the swordfish filets with olive oil and season with salt and pepper. Flame broil the swordfish 3 to 4 minutes a side for a 1-inch thick filet.

4. Move the pasta to a serving platter and top with the barbecued swordfish filets and serve.

Brilliant Oven-Roasted Capon

All out: 3 hr 10 min

Prep: 50 min

Cook: 2 hr 20 min

Yield: 8 servings

Fixings

1 entire (8 pound) capon chicken

Salt and naturally ground dark pepper, to taste

1/4 pound unsalted spread, relaxed

2 lemons, cut down the middle, in addition to 2 tablespoons lemon juice 1/4 cup new slashed herbs, for example, tarragon, thyme or exquisite 1 onion, cut down the middle

4 garlic cloves, crushed

New entire herbs, for example, tarragon leaves, thyme and appetizing sprigs

2 cups water

1/4 cup sherry

Bearings

1.Preheat stove to 450 degrees F. Expel the neck and giblets from the depression and wash the chicken under virus water, all around. Pat dry completely with paper towels. Season the body and depression of the chicken liberally with salt and pepper. In a little bowl, combine the margarine, lemon squeeze and slashed herbs. Rub the herbed spread everywhere throughout the chicken. Put the lemon parts, onion, garlic and entire herbs inside the winged creature. Tie the legs together with kitchen twine to help hold its shape.

2.Spot the chicken, bosom side down, on a V-rack in a broiling container. Cooking the chicken on a rack helps make its skin fresh and shields it from adhering to the base of the skillet. Pour water in the simmering container to keep the fat drippings from consuming and smoking.

3.Cook the chicken for around 20 minutes, at that point cautiously turn the feathered creature over bosom side up. It is ideal to remove the container from the broiler, close the stove entryway to keep up the temperature, and pivot the chicken on the counter. Season the chicken done with the container drippings. Turn the warmth down to 375 degrees F and return the skillet to the broiler. Keep on simmering until a moment read thermometer embedded into the thickest piece of the thigh peruses 165 degrees to 170 degrees F, rely on this taking around 2 hours. Evacuate the chicken to a platter and let represent 15 minutes so the juices settle over into the meat before cutting.

4.In the mean time, pour the drippings from the cooking container into a sauce separator or estimating cup to let the fat ascent to the top. Skim and dispose of the fat at that point return the skillet squeezes back in the simmering dish. Spot the cooking skillet over the stove over medium warmth. Include the sherry and deglaze, scraping up the cooked bits from the base of the dish. Season with salt and pepper, and present with chicken.

Superbly Crunchy Slaw

Absolute: 1 hr 6 min

Prep: 6 min

Dormant: 1 hr

Yield: 4 to 6 servings

Fixings

1/4 little red cabbage, destroyed, around 2 cups

1/3 napa cabbage, destroyed, around 2 cups

2 medium carrots, stripped and ground

1 fennel bulb, meagerly cut

1 Belgian endive skewer, meagerly cut

1/2 cup dried cranberries

1/2 cup toasted pine nuts or pistachio nuts

1/2 cups plain yogurt

2 tablespoons harsh cream

3 tablespoons maple syrup or nectar

1 tablespoon lemon juice

2 cloves garlic, minced

1 teaspoon fit salt

1/4 teaspoon naturally ground dark pepper

1/3 cup slashed chives

Headings

1.In an enormous bowl, combine the cabbages, carrots, fennel, endive, cranberries and pine nuts. In a little bowl, consolidate the yogurt, harsh cream, maple syrup, lemon juice, garlic, salt, and pepper. Pour the dressing over the vegetables and hurl well until covered.

2.Spread and refrigerate for 60 minutes. Trimming with slashed chives before serving.

Lemon Shakerato

- Complete: 5 min
- Dynamic: 5 min
- **Yield: 1 mixed drink**

Fixings

1/2 cup cold-blend espresso
1 tablespoon agave syrup
1/2 teaspoon ground lemon get-up-and-go

Bearings

1. Consolidate the espresso, agave and lemon pizzazz in a shaker half-loaded up with ice. Shake vivaciously for 30 seconds, until foamy. Void the shaker into a stones glass.

Feline's Broccoli Slaw

Absolute: 10 min

Prep: 10 min

Yield: 12 to 16 servings

Fixings

1/3 cup Dijon mustard

1/2 cup sugar

1/3 cup extra-virgin olive oil

3 tablespoons hot sauce

1 teaspoon celery seeds

Genuine salt

Crisply ground dark pepper

2 bundles broccoli slaw

Bearings

1.In a huge bowl, whisk together the mustard and the sugar. Gradually include the rest of the elements for the dressing, proceeding to whisk. Include the broccoli slaw and blend completely.

Container Seared Barramundi with "Caruru"

- All out: 3 hr
- Prep: 45 min
- Idle: 45 min
- Cook: 1 hr 30 min
- **Yield: 4 servings**

Fixings

8 smoked shrimp, cleaved, and shells held

Squeeze salt

1 red onion, diced

4 cloves garlic, fragmented

1 chile, minced

2 tablespoons ground ginger

1 stalk lemongrass, minced

2 to 3 tablespoons margarine, in addition to 2 tablespoons spread

1 red pepper, diced

1 cup slashed okra

2 tomatoes, diced

1 bundle cilantro, leaves cleaved, in addition to extra sprigs for enhancement

1 lime, squeezed

1/2 cup squashed cashews

Oil, for burning

4 (5-ounce) barramundi filets, skin on (may substitute ocean bass or halibut)
Headings

1.Preheat the broiler to 500 degrees F.

2.Toast the shrimp shells in a dry pan over medium-low heat until fragrant and shading has created. Spread the shells with water, include a touch of salt, and stew for 45 minutes over low heat, to shape a stock. Strain the stock through a sifter and put in a safe spot.

3.In a huge pot over low heat, sweat the onion, garlic, chile, ginger, and lemongrass in 2 to 3 tablespoons margarine for 2 minutes. Include the red pepper and sweat for 1 moment more. Include the okra and shrimp stock. Stew the blend for 30 minutes, altering the flavoring as wanted. Overlay in the tomatoes, slashed cilantro, staying 2 tablespoons margarine, lime juice, and cashews. Expel from warmth and hold.

4.Warmth an enormous broiler safe skillet over medium-high heat. Add enough oil to daintily coat the base of the skillet, and let oil heat. Include the fish, skin side down, and burn for 3 minutes. At that point place the skillet in the broiler and dish the fish for a few minutes, or until it arrives at your ideal degree of doneness.

5.Gap the saved stew blend among 4 dishes, and top each with 1 fish filet, skin side up. Enhancement with cilantro sprigs.

Berries with Spiced Cream

- Complete: 10 min
- Dynamic: 10 min
- **Yield: 4 servings**

Fixings

1/2 cup sharp cream or crème fraiche

1/8 teaspoon ground cinnamon

1 cup blueberries

1 cup raspberries

1/4 cup light dark colored sugar

1/2 cup cut almonds, toasted
Bearings

1.Combine the sharp cream and cinnamon in a little bowl. Separation the blueberries and raspberries among 4 roadster glasses or little bowls. Top each presenting with a bit of spiced sharp cream, 1 tablespoon dark colored sugar and a decent sprinkling of toasted almonds.

Atlantic Beach Pie

- Absolute: 4 hr 25 min (incorporates cooling and chilling time)
- Dynamic: 25 min
- **Yield: 8 servings**

Fixings

Covering:

2 1/2 cups shellfish wafers

3 tablespoons sugar

1/2 cup (1 stick) unsalted spread, liquefied

1 tablespoon crisply ground lemon get-up-and-go

Filling:

One 14-ounce can improved consolidated milk

4 enormous egg yolks

1/2 cup crisp lemon juice

Crisp whipped cream, for serving

Naturally ground lemon get-up-and-go, for serving
Headings

1. For the outside layer: Preheat stove to 350 degrees F.

2. Add the saltines and sugar to a nourishment processor and heartbeat a couple of times. Include the dissolved spread and lemon get-up-and-go, at that point beat until the scraps look like wet sand, around 30 seconds. Press piece blend equitably into the base and up the sides of a 8-inch pie skillet, at that point chill for in any event 15 minutes. Heat the hull until the

edges begin to darker, 15 to 17 minutes. Let cool somewhat.

3. For the filling: Add the dense milk and egg yolks to a medium bowl and rush until the yolks are joined. Include the lemon squeeze and speed until completely consolidated, another 1 to 2 minutes. Immerse your readied pie shell and prepare until the filling has almost set in the inside, 20 to 25 minutes. Cool to room temperature, at that point chill in the icebox for in any event 2 hours.

4. Top with whipped cream and newly ground lemon pizzazz and serve

Flame broiled Mahi-Mahi, Ceviche-Style

- Absolute: 2 hr 18 min
- Prep: 10 min
- Dormant: 2 hr
- Cook: 8 min
- **Yield: 4 servings**

Fixings

4 skinless mahi-mahi filets, roughly 2 pounds

2 teaspoons legitimate salt

1/2 cup diced red onion

1/4 cup newly crushed lime juice

1/4 cup newly pressed squeezed orange

1 tablespoon minced jalapeno

1/4 cup dull dark colored sugar, stuffed

1/4 cup tequila

1 tablespoon olive oil

1/4 cup newly hacked cilantro leaves
Bearings

1.Rub the filets with legitimate salt and put in a safe spot. In a non-receptive bowl, consolidate the onion, lime juice, squeezed orange, jalapeno, sugar and tequila. Blend to break up the sugar, and add the filets to the bowl. Marinate in the fridge for 2 hours, turning the filets once following 60 minutes. Expel the filets from the marinade and put it in a safe spot. Pat the filets dry with paper towels and daintily coat with the olive oil.

2.Warmth a flame broil to high and spot the filets over direct heat until they are simply cooked through - obscure at the middle yet wet, around 3 to 4 minutes for every side. While the fish is barbecuing, move the saved marinade to a pan and warmth until it is decreased to around 3/4 cup. Utilizing tongs, evacuate the filets to serving plates and separation sauce similarly among them. Top with the cilantro.

www.ingramcontent.com/pod-product-compliance
Lightning Source LLC
Chambersburg PA
CBHW071829080526
44589CB00012B/962